Textbook of Neonatal Resuscitation, *4th Edition*

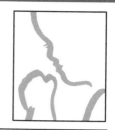

P9-BZL-360

EDITOR
John Kattwinkel, MD, FAAP

EDUCATIONAL DESIGN EDITOR
Jerry Short, PhD

ASSOCIATE EDITORS
Susan Niermeyer, MD, FAAP
Susan E. Denson, MD, FAAP
Jeanette Zaichkin, RNC, MN

NRP Steering Committee Members 1999–2000
Waldemar Carlo, MD, FAAP, Cochair
Susan Niermeyer, MD, FAAP, Cochair
David Boyle, MD, FAAP
Jay P. Goldsmith, MD, FAAP
Jeffrey Perlman, MB, ChB, FAAP
Thomas E. Wiswell, MD, FAAP

NRP Steering Committee Members 1998–1999
Waldemar Carlo, MD, FAAP, Cochair
Susan Niermeyer, MD, FAAP, Cochair
David Boyle, MD, FAAP
Susan E. Denson, MD, FAAP
Martha D. Mullett, MD, FAAP
Jeffrey Perlman, MB, ChB, FAAP

Liaison Representatives 1998–2000
Luis Curet, MD
    American College of Obstetricians and Gynecologists
Barbara Nightengale, RNC, NNP
    National Association of Neonatal Nurses
Michael Speer, MD, FAAP
    AAP Committee on Fetus and Newborn
Alfonso J. Solimano, MD, FRCPC
    Heart and Stroke Foundation of Canada

MANAGING EDITOR
Wendy Simon, MA

MEDICAL ILLUSTRATOR
Lauren Shavell

Based on original text by
Ronald S. Bloom, MD, FAAP
Catherine Cropley, RN, MN

Fourth edition
Third edition, 1994
Second edition, 1990
First edition, 1987

Library of Congress Catalog Card No. 00-131686

ISBN 1-58110-056-6

NRP101

The material is made available as part of the professional education programs of the American Academy of Pediatrics
and the American Heart Association. No endorsement of any product or service should be inferred or is intended.
The Academy has made every effort to ensure that contributors to the Neonatal Resuscitation Program materials
are knowledgeable authorities in their fields. Readers are nevertheless advised that the statements and opinions
expressed are provided as guidelines and should not be construed as official policy of the American Academy of
Pediatrics or the American Heart Association. The recommendations in this publication or the accompanying
materials do not indicate an exclusive course of treatment. Variations, taking into account individual
circumstances, nature of medical oversight, and local protocols, may be appropriate. The American
Academy of Pediatrics and the American Heart Association disclaim any liability or responsibility
for the consequences of any actions taken in the reliance on these statements or opinions.

Acknowledgments

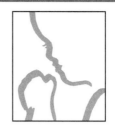

The committee would like to express thanks to the following editors and contributors to the multimedia CD-ROM:

Editors
- Dana A. V. Braner, MD
- Susan E. Denson, MD, FAAP
- Laura M. Ibsen, MD, FAAP

Contributors
- Neil Finer, MD, FAAP
- Joseph Gilhooley, MD
- Susan Niermeyer, MD, FAAP
- Joseph Zennel, MD, FAAP
- Richard Hodo
- Susanna Lai

The committee would like to express thanks to the following consultants and contributors to this textbook:

American Academy of Pediatrics Committee on Fetus and Newborn
American Heart Association, Emergency Cardiac Care Committee, Subcommittee on Pediatric Resuscitation
International Liaison Committee on Resuscitation, Pediatric Working Group
St Mary's Hospital, Clayton, MO
   William Keenan, MD, FAAP
The Media Lab at Doernbecher Children's Hospital
   Dana A. V. Braner, MD
   Laura M. Ibsen, MD, FAAP
University of California, San Diego, San Diego, CA
   Neil Finer, MD, FAAP

AAP Life Support Staff
   Peggy Hecht, MS
   Linda Lipinsky
   Bonnie Molnar
   Becky Shabec
   Wendy Simon, MA
   Shelia Valadez

AAP Marketing and Publications Staff
   Linda Diamond
   Sandi King
   Jill Rubino

The committee would like to express thanks to the following reviewers of this textbook:

Leighton Hill, MD, FAAP
William Keenan, MD, FAAP
Vinay Nadkarni, MD, FAAP
Arno Zaritsky, MD, FAAP

NRP Education Planning Group
   Gary M. Weiner, MD, FAAP
   Linda M. Miller, RN, BSN, MEd
   Margaret A. Putman, MSN, NNP
   Shirley E. Scott, MSN
   Connie K. Styons, RN, MSN, NNP
   Elizabeth B. Turney, MSN
   Brenda Walker, RNC

Associated Education Materials for the *Textbook of Neonatal Resuscitation, 4th Edition*
Cases in Neonatal Resuscitation: Translating Knowledge and Skills Into Practice (video)
   Susan Niermeyer, MD, FAAP, Editor
Instructor's Manual for Neonatal Resuscitation, Jeanette Zaichkin, RNC, MN, Editor
NRP Medication Wall Chart, Code Cart Card, and *Pocket Card,* David Boyle, MD, FAAP, Editor
NRP Slide Presentation Kit, Jay P. Goldsmith, MD, FAAP, Editor
NRP Written Evaluation Packet, Thomas E. Wiswell, MD, FAAP Editor

Contents

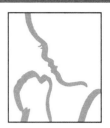

Preface

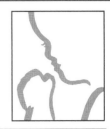

Making the transition from intrauterine to extrauterine life is probably the single most dangerous event that most of us will ever encounter in our lifetimes. Our bodies are required to make more radical physiologic adjustments immediately following birth than they will ever have to do again. The remarkable aspect of birth is that more than 90% of babies make the transition perfectly smoothly, with little to no assistance required. It is for the remaining few percent that the Neonatal Resuscitation Program (NRP) is designed to help. While the percentage requiring assistance may be small, the real number of babies requiring help is substantial because of the large number of births. The implications of not receiving that help can be fatal or associated with problems that can last a lifetime. Skillful resuscitation of a newborn is usually successful, in contrast to resuscitation attempts made on older children or adults. This success can be one of the most gratifying experiences of a health care professional. Learning how to do it well is extremely important.

This textbook has a long history, with many pioneers from both the American Academy of Pediatrics (AAP) and the American Heart Association (AHA) responsible for its evolution. National guidelines for resuscitation of adults were initially recommended in 1966 by the National Academy of Sciences. In 1978, a Working Group on Pediatric Resuscitation was formed by the AHA Emergency Cardiac Care Committee. It quickly concluded that resuscitation of newborns required a different emphasis than resuscitation of adults, with a focus on ventilation rather than cardiac defibrillation being paramount. The formal specialty of neonatology was evolving about that time and, by 1985, the Academy and the AHA expressed a joint commitment to developing a training program aimed at teaching the principles of neonatal resuscitation. The pioneering leaders of this effort were George Peckham and Leon Chameides. A committee was convened to determine the appropriate format for the program and the material written by Ron Bloom and Cathy Cropley was selected to serve as the model for the new NRP textbook.

Pediatric leaders such as Bill Keenan, Errol Alden, Ron Bloom, and John Raye developed a strategy for disseminating the NRP. The strategy first involved training a national faculty that was to consist of at least one physician-nurse team from each state. National faculty training seminars were held and the national faculty, in turn, conducted regional seminars within their respective states. The regional trainers then trained hospital-based instructors and, by the end of 1998, more than 1 million health care providers had been trained in the techniques of neonatal resuscitation.

The science behind the program has also undergone significant evolution. While the ABCD (Airway, Breathing, Circulation, Drugs) principles of resuscitation have been standard for several decades, the details of how and when to accomplish each of the steps and what to do differently for newborns versus older children or adults have required constant evaluation and change.

The AHA has addressed this evaluation process by conducting periodic International Cardiopulmonary Resuscitation and Emergency Cardiac Care (CPR-ECC) conferences every 5 to 8 years to establish guidelines for resuscitation of all age groups and for all causes of cardiopulmonary arrest. The Academy formally joined that process in 1992 for development of the guidelines for resuscitation of children and newborns.

The most recent CPR-ECC conference was held in Dallas in February 2000, and was preceded by a September 1999 Evidence Evaluation conference, which was designed to collect as much published evidence as possible for the February deliberations. The contents of this textbook are based on the recommendations developed at the Guidelines-2000 conference and the document included in the Appendix is the report of the neonatal portion of that conference. For a review of the evidence behind the pages, you are encouraged to consult this document. The next Guidelines conference will be held in 2005. At that time it is likely that some of the recommendations contained in this textbook will change. The Academy has established an NRP Steering Committee consisting of experts with special interest in neonatal resuscitation.

The Steering Committee is responsible for translating the Guidelines into care practices, for determining the structure and implementation strategy for the NRP, for evaluating the science of neonatal resuscitation on an ongoing basis, and for formulating the appropriate questions to be addressed at the next CPR-ECC conference. There is also a dedicated staff at the NRP office housed at the AAP headquarters near Chicago that is available to address any questions you may have about the process and to bring controversies and suggestions about either the science or the process to the attention of the Steering Committee.

The current textbook has undergone some rather significant changes. I hope that those of you who were first trained using the original textbook will not be put off by these changes. Jerry Short, an authority in educational design, has worked closely with me to structure the material to be educationally sound while still relevant and comfortable to the practicing clinician. We have opened many of the lessons with clinical scenarios intended to illustrate the concepts and skills covered in the respective lessons. We have tried to structure the book to be readable to clinicians with all levels of expertise, from the novice to the neonatologist. We have added a list of "Key Points" at the end of each lesson as a review for the novice and as a means to make the identification of new content more efficient for the experienced resuscitator. In addition, we have tried to simplify some of the guidelines that had proved to be confusing, such as the heart rate levels at which one initiates chest compressions or gives medications.

Probably the most significant change involves our recommendations about how to evaluate the baby and how to implement the resuscitation steps. The original NRP presented a "hierarchical" approach: first evaluate and treat the respirations, then evaluate and treat the heart rate, and then evaluate and treat the color. After much discussion, it was the consensus of the Steering Committee that, during a real resuscitation, experts use a more "integrated" approach, in which the baby's risk factors, appearance, and color are evaluated simultaneously as the initial steps of resuscitation are administered. Then respirations, heart rate, and color are evaluated again as a near-simultaneous process while deciding what further intervention is required.

You will find that the same six topics from the original textbook are presented in sequential chapters and you will find some of the same text from the excellent original Bloom and Cropley edition. However, throughout the revised program, we have tried to emphasize this concept of integrated assessment and actions. Finally, we have added a new chapter to address some of the more subjective aspects of neonatal resuscitation: What do you do when the basic steps are not working or you are resuscitating outside of the hospital delivery area? How should you care for the baby after resuscitation? And the very important question of when is it appropriate to stop or perhaps not even start resuscitation of a newly born baby? This latter topic cannot, of course, be addressed adequately in a few pages. But many of us felt that the topic was far too important not to be covered to some degree.

There also are some additional formats that we introduce with this first edition of the new century. We hope that the CD-ROM and the video will make the written concepts more realistic and understandable and will make the learning more enjoyable to those with an interest in the new media formats. Conversely, it is our intent that the textbook alone will be sufficient to convey all the essential content.

However you decide to learn the factual material, your demonstration sessions with an instructor using the Performance Checklists and your opportunity to practice with colleagues functioning as a team are probably the most important activities associated with the NRP.

I do not want to close this preface without recognizing the many individuals that have collaborated to produce the textbook. The vast majority of these individuals have volunteered their time, and even those few who have been salaried have worked well beyond the limits of their job descriptions. I have already mentioned Dr Jerry Short, whose educational design concepts are evident throughout the pages. Wendy Simon is solely responsible for making all the components come together cohesively and on schedule. Linda Lipinsky negotiated the integration of AHA and AAP interests. All the members of the NRP Steering Committee spent tireless hours determining the content. The many members of the AHA Pediatric Subcommittee, under the leadership of Vinay Nadkarni, Bob Berg, and Arno Zaritsky, worked hard to ensure the content between the NRP and the other AHA programs convey similar messages. Lauren Shavell worked diligently at drawing the new figures, and Dana Braner created the photographs and managed to coordinate the

timetable for production of the CD-ROM and video with the deadlines set for the textbook. Susan Denson, Bill Keenan, and Jeanette Zaichkin, were superb collaborators in preparation of the figures, text, and Performance Checklists. Jill Rubino from the Academy and FG Stoddard from the AHA were wonderfully patient and instructive copy editors. Susan Niermeyer probably has been the most important figure in the recent history of the NRP project. Her primary authorship of the Guidelines-2000 document, her superb critiques of the many drafts of the textbook, and her expert knowledge of how to teach effectively have been invaluable. The concept of the importance of integrated assessment and action was as much hers as anyone's. The final product of the NRP is a reflection of an effort by many individuals working together as an integrated team — much as is required for the successful resuscitation of a compromised newborn. Please let us know what has been effective and what has not as we begin work on the next edition.

John Kattwinkel, MD

NRP Provider Course Overview

Neonatal Resuscitation Scientific Guidelines

This course is based on the American Academy of Pediatrics (AAP) and American Heart Association's International Guidelines for Emergency Cardiovascular Care of the Newborn. If you are interested in reviewing only the scientific recommendations, please refer to the Appendix where you will find the official neonatal resuscitation guidelines. You also should refer to these pages if you have questions about the rationale for the current program recommendations.

Level of Responsibility

The standard-length Neonatal Resuscitation Program (NRP) provider course consists of seven lessons. However, you will need to work through only those lessons appropriate to your level of responsibility. Resuscitation responsibilities vary from hospital to hospital. For example, in some institutions, nurses may be responsible for intubating the newborn, but, in others, the physician or respiratory therapist may do so. The number of lessons you will need to complete depends on your personal level of responsibility.

Before starting the course, you must have a clear idea of your exact responsibilities. If you have any questions about the level of your responsibilities during resuscitation, please consult your instructor or supervisor.

Special Note: Neonatal resuscitation is most effective when performed by a designated and coordinated team. It is important for you to know the neonatal resuscitation responsibilities of team members who are working with you. Periodic practice among team members will facilitate coordinated and effective care of the infant.

Lesson Completion

Successful completion of each lesson requires a passing score on the written evaluation for that lesson as well as successful completion of the performance checklist (for lessons 2 through 6). Upon successful completion of at least lessons 1 through 4, participants are eligible to receive a course completion card. This verification of participation is not issued on the day of the course. Instructors will distribute course completion cards after the course roster is received and processed by the AAP Life Support staff.

Completion Does Not Imply Competence

The Neonatal Resuscitation Program is an educational program that introduces the concepts and basic skills of neonatal resuscitation. **Completion of the program does not imply that an individual has the competence to perform neonatal resuscitation.** Each hospital is responsible for determining the level of competence and qualifications required for someone to assume clinical responsibility for neonatal resuscitation.

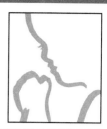

Standard Precautions

The US Centers for Disease Control and Prevention have recommended that standard precautions be taken whenever risk of exposure to blood or bodily fluids is high and the potential infectious status of the patient is unknown, as is certainly the case in neonatal resuscitation.

All fluid products from patients (blood, urine, stool, saliva, vomitus, etc) should be treated as potentially infectious. Gloves should be worn when resuscitating a newborn, and the rescuer should not use his or her mouth to apply suction via a suction device. Mouth-to-mouth resuscitation should be avoided by having a bag-and-mask device always available for use during resuscitation. Masks and protective eyewear or face shields should be worn during procedures that are likely to generate droplets of blood or other bodily fluids. Gowns and aprons should be worn during procedures that will probably generate splashes of blood or other bodily fluids. Delivery rooms must be equipped with resuscitation bags, masks, laryngoscopes, endotracheal tubes, mechanical suction devices, and the necessary protective shields.

Textbook of Neonatal Resuscitation, 4th Edition, Multimedia CD-ROM

The new *Textbook of Neonatal Resuscitation, 4th Edition, Multimedia CD-ROM* is located on the inside back cover of this text. System requirements, and content specifications are located on the inside front cover. In addition to all of the content and illustrations contained in the textbook, the CD-ROM contains dramatic footage of actual resuscitation events, laryngoscopic view of the airway, digitized animation, review questions, and learner-directed interactive video scenarios.

It is up to you to choose whether to learn the NRP content through reading the textbook, viewing the CD-ROM, or a combination of the two. However, the NRP Steering Committee highly encourages learners to make use of all resources available to them. The CD-ROM offers great learning value as it shows real-time video footage of the NRP steps.

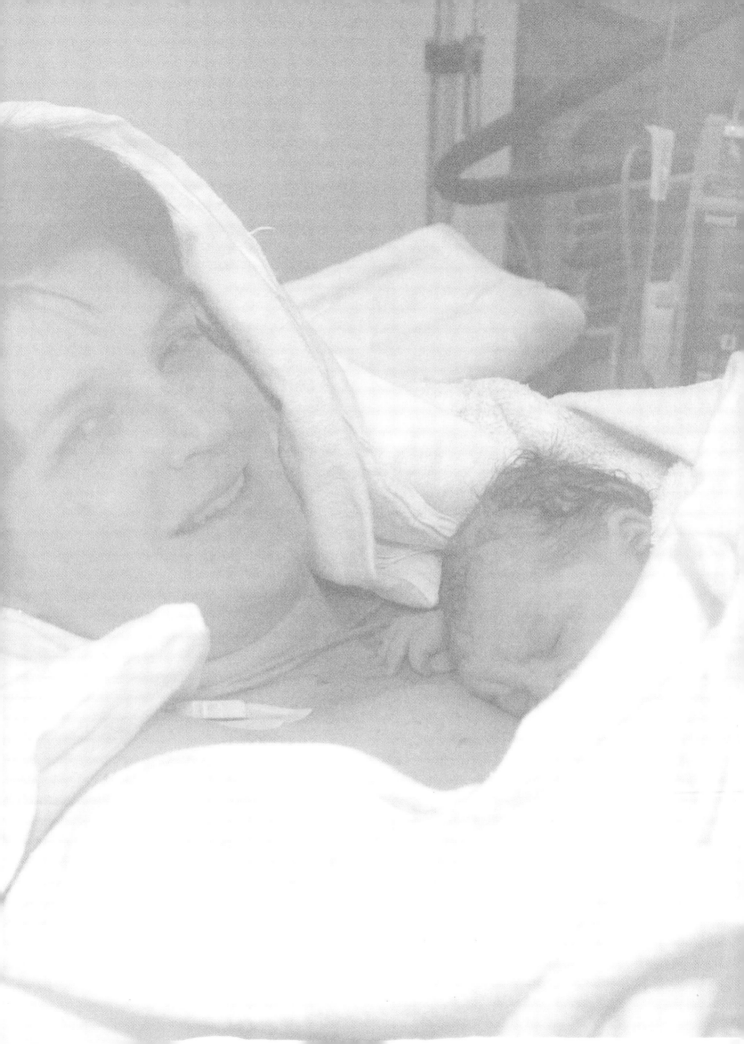

1

Overview and Principles of Resuscitation

The Neonatal Resuscitation Program (NRP) will help you learn how to resuscitate newborns. By studying this book and practicing the skills, you will learn how to be a valuable member of the resuscitation team.

Many concepts and skills are taught in the program. However, the major concept of NRP, which is emphasized throughout the program, is this:

The most important and effective action in neonatal resuscitation is to ventilate the baby's lungs with oxygen.

In Lesson 1 you will learn the

• Changes in physiology that occur when a baby is born

• Flow diagram showing all the steps to follow during resuscitation

• Risk factors that can help predict which babies will require resuscitation

• Equipment and personnel needed to resuscitate a newborn

Why learn neonatal resuscitation?

Birth asphyxia accounts for about 19% of the approximately 5 million neonatal deaths that occur each year worldwide (World Health Organization, 1995). This suggests that the outcomes of more than *1 million newborns* per year might be improved by using the resuscitation techniques taught in this program.

Which babies require resuscitation?

Approximately 10% of newborns require some assistance to begin breathing at birth; about 1% need extensive resuscitative measures to survive. In contrast, at least 90% of newly born babies make the transition from intrauterine to extrauterine life without difficulty. They require little to no assistance initiating spontaneous and regular respirations.

The "ABCs" of resuscitation are the same for babies as for adults. Ensure that the Airway is open and clear. Be sure that there is Breathing, whether spontaneous or assisted. Make certain that there is adequate Circulation of oxygenated blood. Newly born babies are wet following birth and heat loss is great. Therefore, it also is important to maintain body temperature during resuscitation.

The diagram below illustrates the relationship between resuscitation procedures and the number of newly born babies who need them. At the top are the procedures needed by all newborns. At the bottom are procedures needed by very few.

ABCs of resuscitation

Airway
(position and clear)

Breathing
(stimulate to breathe)

Circulation
(assess heart rate and color)

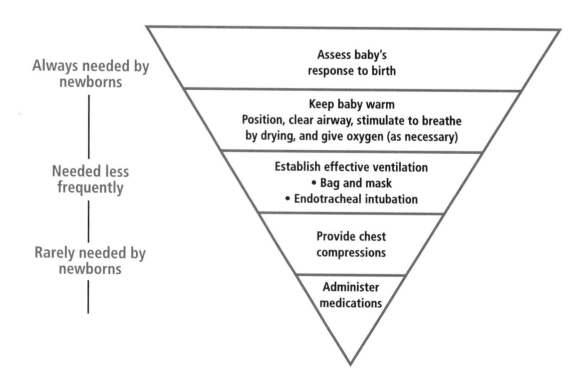

Always needed by newborns

Needed less frequently

Rarely needed by newborns

Assess baby's response to birth

Keep baby warm
Position, clear airway, stimulate to breathe by drying, and give oxygen (as necessary)

Establish effective ventilation
• Bag and mask
• Endotracheal intubation

Provide chest compressions

Administer medications

✔ Check yourself!

(The answers are in the preceding section and at the end of the lesson.)

1. About _____ million babies' lives per year worldwide could be saved by proper resuscitation.

2. About _____% of newborns will require some assistance to begin regular breathing.

3. About _____% of newborns will require extensive resuscitation to survive.

4. Chest compressions and medications are (rarely) (frequently) needed when resuscitating newborns.

The Neonatal Resuscitation Program is organized in the following way:

Lesson 1: Overview and Principles of Resuscitation

Lesson 2: Initial Steps in Resuscitation

Lesson 3: Use of a Resuscitation Bag and Mask

Lesson 4: Chest Compressions

Lesson 5: Endotracheal Intubation

Lesson 6: Medications

Lesson 7: Special Considerations

You will have many opportunities to practice the steps involved in resuscitation and use the appropriate resuscitation equipment. You will gradually build your proficiency and speed. In addition, you will learn to evaluate a newborn throughout resuscitation and make decisions about what actions to take next.

In the next section, you will learn the basic physiology involved in a baby's transition from intrauterine to extrauterine life. Understanding the physiology involved in breathing and circulation in the newborn will help you understand why prompt resuscitation is so important in saving lives.

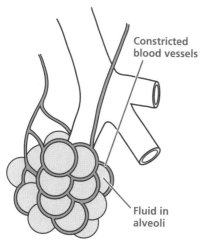

Figure 1.1. Fluid-filled alveoli and constricted blood vessels in the lung before birth

How does a baby receive oxygen before birth?

Oxygen is essential for survival both before birth and after birth. Before birth, all of the oxygen used by a fetus diffuses across the placental membrane from the mother's blood to the baby's blood.

Before birth, only a small fraction of fetal blood passes through the fetal lungs. The fetal lungs do not function as a source for oxygen or as a route to excrete carbon dioxide. Therefore, it is less important for the lungs to be perfused. The fetal lungs are expanded in utero, but the potential air sacs within the lungs (alveoli) are filled with fluid, rather than air. In addition, the blood vessels that perfuse and drain the fetal lungs are markedly constricted (Figure 1.1).

Before birth, most of the blood from the right side of the heart cannot enter the lungs because of the constricted blood vessels in the fetal lungs. Instead, most of this blood flows through the ductus arteriosus into the aorta (Figure 1.2).

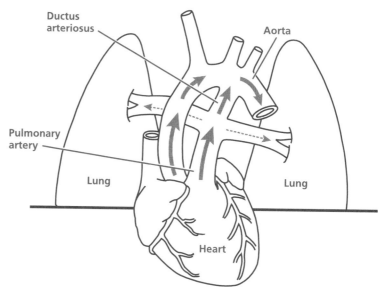

Figure 1.2. Shunting of blood through the ductus arteriosus and away from the lungs before birth

After birth, the newborn will no longer be connected to the placenta and will depend on the lungs as the only source of oxygen. Therefore, over a matter of seconds, the lungs must fill with oxygen, and the blood vessels in the lungs must relax to perfuse the alveoli and to absorb oxygen and carry it to the rest of the body.

What normally happens at birth to allow a baby to get oxygen from the lungs?

Normally, there are three major changes that take place within seconds after birth.

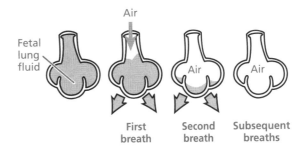

Figure 1.3. Fluid replaced by air in alveoli

1. The **fluid in the alveoli is absorbed** into lung tissue and replaced by air (Figure 1.3). The oxygen in the air is then able to diffuse into the blood vessels that surround the alveoli.

2. The **umbilical arteries and vein are clamped.** This removes the low-resistance placental circuit and increases systemic blood pressure.

3. As a result of the gaseous distention and increased oxygen in the alveoli, the **blood vessels in the lung tissue relax** (Figure 1.4). This relaxation, together with the increased systemic blood pressure, creates a dramatic increase in pulmonary blood flow and a decrease in flow through the ductus arteriosus. The oxygen from the alveoli is absorbed by the increased pulmonary blood flow, and the oxygen-enriched blood returns to the left side of the heart where it is pumped to the tissues of the newborn's body.

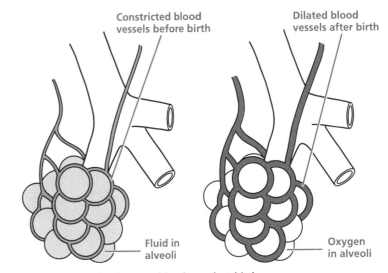

Figure 1.4. Dilation of pulmonary blood vessels at birth

As blood levels of oxygen increase and pulmonary blood vessels relax, the ductus arteriosus begins to constrict. Blood previously diverted through the ductus arteriosus now flows through the lungs, where it picks up more oxygen to transport to tissues throughout the body (Figure 1.5).

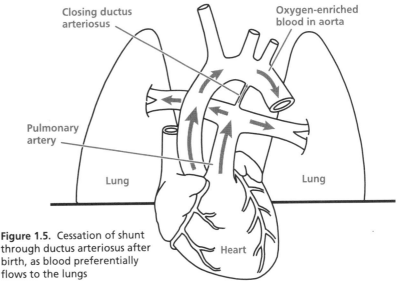

Figure 1.5. Cessation of shunt through ductus arteriosus after birth, as blood preferentially flows to the lungs

At the completion of this normal transition, the baby is breathing air and using his lungs to get oxygen. His initial cries and deep breaths have been strong enough to help move the fluid from his airways. The oxygen and gaseous distention of the lungs are the main stimuli for the pulmonary blood vessels to relax. As adequate oxygen enters the blood, the baby's skin turns from gray/blue to pink.

What can go wrong during transition?

A baby may encounter difficulty before labor, during labor, or after birth. If the difficulty begins in utero, either before or during labor, the problem will usually reflect a compromised blood flow in the placenta or the umbilical cord. The first clinical sign can be a deceleration of the fetal heart rate. Problems encountered after birth are more likely to involve the baby's airway. The following are some of the problems that may disrupt normal transition:

- The baby may not breathe sufficiently to force fluid from the alveoli or foreign material, such as meconium, may block air from entering the alveoli. As a result, the lungs will not fill with air, and oxygen will not be available to blood circulating through the lungs.

- Excessive blood loss may occur, or there may be poor cardiac contractility or bradycardia from hypoxia, so that the expected increase in blood pressure cannot occur (systemic hypotension).

- A lack of oxygen or failure of gaseous distention of the lungs may result in sustained constriction of the pulmonary arterioles. These arterioles may then remain constricted, thus preventing oxygen from reaching body tissues (persistent pulmonary hypertension).

How does a baby respond to an interruption in normal transition?

Normally, newborns will make vigorous efforts to pull air into their lungs. This causes fetal lung fluid to move out of the alveoli and into the surrounding lung tissue. This also brings oxygen to the pulmonary arterioles and causes the arterioles to relax. If this sequence is interrupted, the pulmonary arterioles can remain constricted, and the systemic arterial blood may not become oxygenated.

In addition to persistent vasoconstriction of the pulmonary vasculature, the arterioles in the bowels, kidneys, muscles, and skin will constrict, while blood flow to the heart and brain is preserved. This redistribution of blood flow helps preserve function of the vital organs. However, if oxygen deprivation continues, myocardial function and cardiac output deteriorate, and blood flow to all organs is reduced. The consequence of this lack of adequate blood perfusion and tissue oxygenation can be brain damage, damage to other organs, or death.

The compromised baby may exhibit one or more of the following clinical findings:

- Cyanosis from insufficient oxygen in the blood

- Bradycardia from insufficient delivery of oxygen to the heart muscle or brain stem

- Low blood pressure from insufficient oxygen to the heart muscle, blood loss, or insufficient blood return from the placenta before or during birth

- Depression of respiratory drive from insufficient oxygen delivery to the brain
- Poor muscle tone from insufficient oxygen delivery to the brain and muscles

Many of these same symptoms may also occur in other conditions, such as infection or hypoglycemia, or if the baby's respiratory efforts have been depressed by depressant medications given to the mother before birth.

How can you tell if a newborn had in utero or perinatal compromise?

Laboratory studies have shown that respirations are the first vital sign to cease when a newborn is deprived of oxygen. After an initial period of rapid attempts to breathe, there is a period of *primary apnea* (Figure 1.6), during which stimulation, such as drying or slapping the feet, will cause a resumption of breathing.

However, if oxygen deprivation continues, the baby will make several attempts to gasp and then will enter a period of *secondary apnea* (Figure 1.6). During secondary apnea, stimulation will *not* restart the baby's breathing. Assisted ventilation must be provided for the process to reverse.

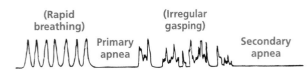

Figure 1.6. Primary and secondary apnea

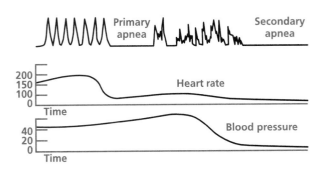

Figure 1.7. Heart rate and blood pressure changes during apnea

 If a baby does not begin breathing immediately after being stimulated, he or she is likely in secondary apnea and will require positive-pressure ventilation. Continued stimulation will not help.

Heart rate begins to fall at about the same time that the baby enters primary apnea. Blood pressure is usually maintained until the onset of secondary apnea (unless blood loss has resulted in an earlier onset of hypotension) (Figure 1.7).

Most of the time, the baby will be presented to you somewhere in the middle of the sequence described above. Often, the compromising event will have started before or during labor. Therefore, at the time of birth, it will be difficult to determine how long the baby has been compromised. The heart rate and respiratory response to stimulation may help you estimate how recently the event began. As a general rule, the longer a baby has been compromised, the longer it will take for vital signs to recover.

Check yourself!

(The answers are in the preceding section and at the end of the lesson.)

5. Before birth, the alveoli in a baby's lungs are (collapsed) (expanded) and filled with (fluid) (air).

6. At birth, a baby's strong breathing causes _____ to be absorbed from the lungs and replaced with _____ .

7. The oxygen in the baby's lungs then causes the pulmonary arterioles to (relax) (constrict) so that the oxygen can be absorbed from the alveoli and distributed to all organs.

8. If a baby does not begin breathing in response to stimulation, you should assume he is in _____ apnea, and you should provide _____ .

9. If sufficient oxygen does not get to the baby's blood and he enters the stage of secondary apnea, he will be (blue) (pink), his heart rate will (rise) (fall), and his blood pressure will (rise) (fall).

The resuscitation flow diagram

This flow diagram describes all of the NRP resuscitation procedures. The diagram begins with the birth of the baby. Each resuscitation step is shown in a block. Below each block is a decision point to help you decide if you need to proceed to the next step.

Study the diagram as you read the description of each step and decision point. This diagram will be repeated in later lessons. Use it to help you remember the steps involved in a resuscitation.

Assessment Block. At the time of birth, you should ask yourself five questions about the newborn. These questions are shown in the Assessment block of the diagram. If any answer is "No," you should continue to the initial steps of resuscitation.

A **Block A (Airway).** These are the initial steps you take to establish an Airway and begin resuscitating a newborn.

- Provide warmth.
- Position the baby's head to open the airway; clear the airway as necessary.
- Dry the baby, stimulate the baby to breath, and reposition the baby's head to open the airway.
- Give oxygen as necessary.

Note how quickly you evaluate the baby and take the initial steps. As the time line shows, you should complete these blocks in about 30 seconds.

Evaluation of Block A. You evaluate the newborn after about 30 seconds. If the newborn is not breathing (has apnea) or has a heart rate of less than 100 beats per minute (bpm), you proceed to Block B.

B **Block B (Breathing).** You assist the baby's Breathing by providing positive-pressure ventilation with a bag and mask for about 30 seconds.

Evaluation of Block B. After about 30 seconds of ventilation, you evaluate the newborn again. If the heart rate is below 60 bpm, you proceed to Block C.

C **Block C (Circulation).** You support Circulation by starting chest compressions while continuing positive-pressure ventilation.

Evaluation of Block C. After about 30 seconds of chest compressions, you evaluate the newborn again. If the heart rate is still below 60 bpm, you proceed to Block D.

D **Block D (Drug).** You administer epinephrine as you continue positive-pressure ventilation and chest compressions.

Evaluation of Block D. If the heart rate remains below 60 bpm, the actions in Blocks C and D are continued and repeated. This is indicated by the curved arrow.

Birth

APPROXIMATE TIME

30 SECONDS

- Clear of meconium?
- Breathing or crying?
- Good muscle tone?
- Color pink?
- Term gestation?

Assessment

No

- Provide warmth
- Position; clear airway* (as necessary)
- Dry, stimulate, reposition
- Give O$_2$ (as necessary)

A

30 SECONDS

- Evaluate respirations, heart rate, and color

Evaluation

Apnea   *or HR<100*

- Provide positive-pressure ventilation*

B

Evaluation

HR<60   *HR>60*

30 SECONDS

- Provide positive-pressure ventilation*
- Administer chest compressions

C

Evaluation

HR<60

- Administer epinephrine*

D

*Endotracheal intubation may be considered at several steps.

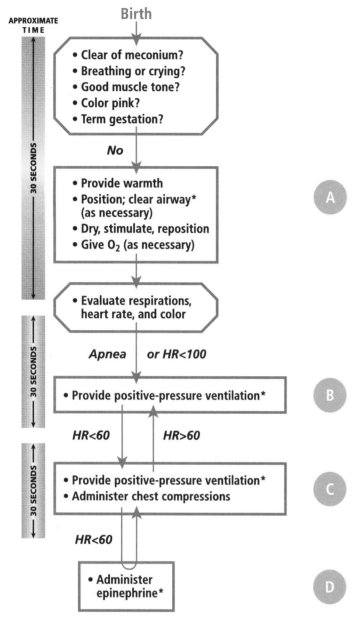

APPROXIMATE
TIME

Birth

30 SECONDS

- Clear of meconium?
- Breathing or crying?
- Good muscle tone?
- Color pink?
- Term gestation?

No

- Provide warmth
- Position; clear airway* (as necessary)
- Dry, stimulate, reposition
- Give O₂ (as necessary)

A

- Evaluate respirations, heart rate, and color

Apnea | *or HR<100*

30 SECONDS

- Provide positive-pressure ventilation*

B

HR<60 | *HR>60*

30 SECONDS

- Provide positive-pressure ventilation*
- Administer chest compressions

C

HR<60

- Administer epinephrine*

D

*Endotracheal intubation may be considered at several steps.

When the heart rate improves and rises above 60 bpm, chest compressions are stopped. Positive-pressure ventilation is continued until the heart rate is above 100 bpm and the baby is breathing.

Please note the following important points about the flow diagram:

- There are two heart rates to remember: 60 bpm and 100 bpm. In general, a heart rate below 60 bpm indicates that additional resuscitation steps are needed. A heart rate above 100 bpm usually indicates that resuscitation procedures can be stopped.

- The asterisks (*) in the flow diagram indicate points at which endotracheal intubation may be needed. These points will be described in later lessons.

- The time line beside the flow diagram indicates how quickly resuscitation proceeds from step to step. Do not continue a step beyond about 30 seconds if a newborn shows no improvement. Instead, proceed to the next step in the flow diagram.

- The primary actions in neonatal resuscitation are aimed at getting oxygen into the baby's lungs (Blocks A and B). Once this has been accomplished, heart rate, blood pressure, and pulmonary blood flow will usually improve spontaneously. However, if blood and tissue oxygen levels have become extremely low, cardiac output may have to be assisted by chest compressions and epinephrine (Blocks C and D) in order for blood to reach the lungs to pick up oxygen.

Now take time to become familiar with the flow diagram, and learn the order of steps that will be presented in the following lessons. Also learn the heart rates you use to decide if the next step is needed.

Look at the color photographs in the center of the book (Center Pages A through D). Figure A-1 has all the characteristics of a vigorous baby born at term and needs only routine care. Figure B-2 has poor muscle tone and color and requires resuscitation.

How do you prioritize your actions?

A very important cycle repeated throughout resuscitation consists of evaluating the newborn, deciding what action to take, and taking action. Then repeat the evaluation using the new vital signs as the basis for more decisions and further actions.

Evaluation is based primarily on the following three signs:

- Respirations
- Heart rate
- Color

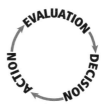

This evaluation-decision-action symbol will appear throughout the text to signal particularly important concepts.

An exclamation mark will be placed next to items that are particularly important for you to remember.

Why is the Apgar score *not* used during resuscitation?

The Apgar score is an objective method of quantifying the newborn's condition and is useful for conveying information about the newborn's overall status and response to resuscitation. However, resuscitation must be initiated before the score is assigned. Therefore, *the Apgar score is not used to determine the need for resuscitation, what resuscitation steps are necessary, or when to use them.* The three signs that you will use to decide how and when to resuscitate (respirations, heart rate, and color) do form part of the score. Two additional elements (muscle tone and reflex irritability) reflect neurologic status.

The Apgar score is normally assigned at 1 minute and again at 5 minutes of age. When the 5-minute score is less than 7, additional scores should be assigned every 5 minutes for up to 20 minutes. Elements of the Apgar score are described in the Appendix at the end of this lesson.

How do you prepare for a resuscitation?

At every birth, you should be prepared to resuscitate a newborn because the need for resuscitation can come as a complete surprise. For this reason, every birth should be attended by at least one person skilled in neonatal resuscitation whose sole responsibility is management of the newborn. Additional personnel will be needed if more complex resuscitation is anticipated.

With careful consideration of risk factors, more than half of all newborns who will need resuscitation can be identified prior to birth. If you anticipate the possible need for neonatal resuscitation, you can

• Recruit additional skilled personnel to be present.

• Prepare the necessary equipment.

What risk factors are associated with the need for neonatal resuscitation?

Review this list of risk factors.
Consider having a copy readily available in the labor and delivery areas.

Antepartum Factors

Maternal diabetes	Post-term gestation
Pregnancy-induced hypertension	Multiple gestation
Chronic hypertension	Size-dates discrepancy
Anemia or isoimmunization	Drug therapy, eg,
Previous fetal or neonatal death	Lithium carbonate
Bleeding in second or third trimester	Magnesium
Maternal infection	Adrenergic-blocking drugs
Maternal cardiac, renal, pulmonary,	Maternal substance abuse
thyroid, or neurologic disease	Fetal malformation
Polyhydramnios	Diminished fetal activity
Oligohydramnios	No prenatal care
Premature rupture of membranes	Age <16 or >35 years

Intrapartum Factors

Emergency cesarean section	Fetal bradycardia
Forceps or vacuum-assisted delivery	Non-reassuring fetal heart rate patterns
Breech or other abnormal presentation	Use of general anesthesia
Premature labor	Uterine tetany
Precipitous labor	Narcotics administered to mother
Chorioamnionitis	within 4 hours of delivery
Prolonged rupture of membranes	Meconium-stained amniotic fluid
(>18 hours before delivery)	Prolapsed cord
Prolonged labor (>24 hours)	Abruptio placentae
Prolonged second stage of labor (>2 hours)	Placenta previa

Why are premature babies at higher risk?

Many of these risk factors may result in a baby being born preterm. Premature babies have anatomical and physiological characteristics that are quite different from babies born at term. Some of these characteristics are

- Their lungs may be deficient in surfactant and, therefore, may be more difficult to ventilate.

- Their thin, permeable skin, large surface-area-to-body-mass ratio, and lack of subcutaneous fat make them more likely to lose heat.

- They are more likely to be born with an infection.

- Their brains have very fragile capillaries that may bleed during periods of stress.

These and other unique characteristics present special challenges during resuscitation of premature babies. When special considerations for premature babies are indicated, they will be brought to your attention during the program.

Check yourself!

(The answers are in the preceding section and at the end of the lesson.)

10. Complete the missing parts of the chart.
    A. Apnea or heart rate < _____
    B. Provide _____
    C. Heart rate < _____
    D. Provide positive-pressure ventilation and

    _____
    E. Heart rate < _____

11. Resuscitation (should) (should not) be delayed until the 1-minute Apgar score is available.

12. Premature babies may present unique challenges during resuscitation because of
    A. Fragile brain capillaries that may bleed
    B. Lungs deficient in surfactant, making ventilation difficult
    C. Poor temperature control
    D. Higher likelihood of an infection
    E. All of the above

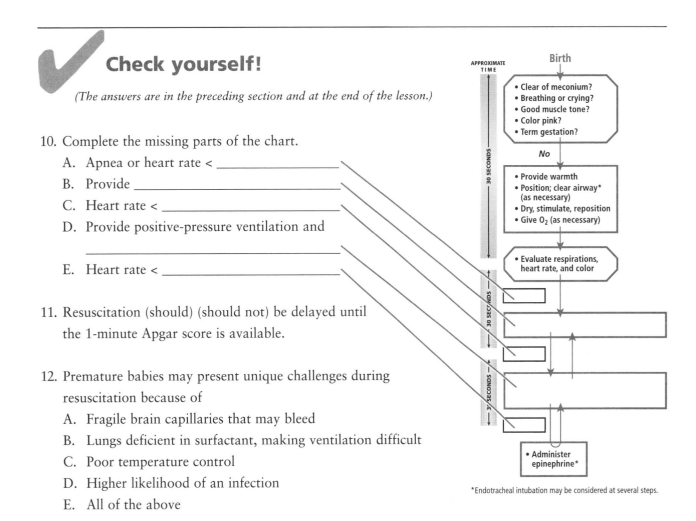

APPROXIMATE TIME

Birth

- Clear of meconium?
- Breathing or crying?
- Good muscle tone?
- Color pink?
- Term gestation?

No

- Provide warmth
- Position; clear airway* (as necessary)
- Dry, stimulate, reposition
- Give O$_2$ (as necessary)

- Evaluate respirations, heart rate, and color

30 SECONDS

30 SECONDS

30 SECONDS

- Administer epinephrine*

*Endotracheal intubation may be considered at several steps.

What personnel should be present at delivery?

At every delivery, there should be at least one person whose primary responsibility is the baby and who is capable of initiating resuscitation. Either that person or someone else who is immediately available should have the skills required to perform a complete resuscitation, including endotracheal intubation and administration of medications. It is not sufficient to have someone "on call" (either at home or in a remote area of the hospital) for newborn resuscitations in the delivery room. When resuscitation is needed, it must be initiated without delay.

If the delivery is anticipated to be high-risk, and thus may require more advanced neonatal resuscitation, at least two persons should be present solely to manage the baby — one with complete resuscitation skills and one or more to assist. The concept of a "resuscitation team," with a specified leader and an identified role for each member, should be the goal. For multiple births, a separate team should be organized for each baby.

For example, a delivery room nurse is present at an uncomplicated birth. This nurse might initially clear the airway, provide tactile stimulation, and evaluate the respirations and heart rate. If the newborn does not respond appropriately, the nurse would initiate bag-and-mask ventilation and call for assistance. A physician, nurse, or respiratory therapist with full resuscitation skills would be in the immediate vicinity and available to intubate the trachea and assist with coordinated chest compressions and ventilation.

In the case of an anticipated high-risk birth, two, three, or even four people with varying degrees of resuscitation skills may be needed at the delivery. One of them, with complete resuscitation skills, would serve as the leader of the team and would probably be the one to position the baby, open the airway, and intubate the trachea if necessary. Two others would assist with positioning, suctioning, drying, and giving oxygen. They could administer positive-pressure ventilation or chest compressions as directed by the leader. A fourth person would be helpful for administering medications and/or documenting the events.

Remember that a birth is associated with much blood and other body fluids, and a neonatal resuscitation provides considerable opportunity for transmission of infectious agents. Be sure that all personnel observe appropriate standard precautions as defined by hospital policy.

What equipment should be available?

All the equipment necessary for a complete resuscitation must be in the delivery room and be fully operational. When a high-risk newborn is expected, appropriate equipment should be ready to use. A complete list of neonatal resuscitation equipment is in the Appendix at the end of this lesson.

What do you do after a resuscitation?

Babies who have required resuscitation are at risk for deterioration after their vital signs have returned to normal. You learned earlier in this lesson that the longer a baby has been compromised, the longer he or she will take to respond to resuscitation efforts. The NRP will refer to the following three levels of post-resuscitation care:

Routine Care: Nearly 90% of newborns are vigorous term babies with no risk factors and clear amniotic fluid. They do not need to be separated from their mothers after birth in order to receive the initial steps of resuscitation. Thermoregulation can be provided by putting the baby directly on the mother's chest, drying, and covering with dry linen. Warmth is maintained by direct skin-to-skin contact with the mother. Clearing of the upper airway can be provided as necessary by wiping the baby's mouth and nose. While the initial steps can be provided in modified form, ongoing observation of breathing, activity, and color must be carried out to determine the need for additional intervention.

Supportive Care: Babies who have prenatal or intrapartum risk factors, have meconium staining of the amniotic fluid or skin, have depressed breathing or activity, and/or are cyanotic will need some degree of resuscitation at birth. These babies should be evaluated and managed initially under a radiant warmer and should receive the initial steps as appropriate. These babies are still at risk for developing problems associated with perinatal compromise and should be evaluated frequently during the immediate neonatal period.

Ongoing Care: Babies who required positive-pressure ventilation or more extensive resuscitation may require ongoing support, are at high risk for recurrent deterioration, and are at high risk for developing subsequent complications of an abnormal transition. These babies generally should be managed in an environment where ongoing evaluation and monitoring are available. Transfer to an intensive care nursery may be necessary.

Birth

- Clear of meconium?
- Breathing or crying?
- Good muscle tone?
- Color pink?
- Term gestation?

Yes →

Routine care
- Provide warmth
- Clear airway
- Dry

No

- Provide warmth
- Position; clear airway* (as necessary)
- Dry, stimulate, reposition
- Give O$_2$ (as necessary)

- Evaluate respirations, heart rate, and color

Breathing
HR>100 & Pink → **Supportive care**

Apnea or *HR<100*

- Provide positive-pressure ventilation*

Ventilating
HR>100 & Pink → **Ongoing care**

HR<60 *HR>60*

- Provide positive-pressure ventilation*
- Administer chest compressions

HR<60

- Administer epinephrine*

*Endotracheal intubation may be considered at several steps.

Lesson 1 Review

(The answers are at the end of the lesson.)

1. About _____ million babies' lives per year worldwide could be saved by proper resuscitation.

2. About _____% of newborns will require some assistance to begin regular breathing.

3. About _____% of newborns will require extensive resuscitation to survive.

4. Chest compressions and medications are (rarely) (frequently) needed when resuscitating newborns.

5. Before birth, the alveoli in a baby's lungs are (collapsed) (expanded) and filled with (fluid) (air).

6. At birth, a baby's strong breathing causes _____ to be absorbed from the lungs and replaced with _____ .

7. The oxygen in the baby's lungs then causes the pulmonary arterioles to (relax) (constrict) so that the oxygen can be absorbed from alveoli and distributed to all organs.

8. If a baby does not begin breathing in response to stimulation, you should assume he is in _____ apnea and you should provide _____ .

9. If sufficient oxygen does not get to the baby's blood and he enters the stage of secondary apnea, he will be (blue) (pink), his heart rate will (rise) (fall), and his blood pressure will (rise) (fall).

Lesson 1 Review — *continued*

(The answers are at the end of the lesson.)

10. Complete the missing parts of the chart.
    A. Apnea or heart rate < _____
    B. Provide _____
    C. Heart rate < _____
    D. Provide positive-pressure ventilation and

    _____
    E. Heart rate < _____

11. Resuscitation (should) (should not) be delayed until the 1-minute Apgar score is available.

12. Premature babies may present unique challenges during resuscitation because of
    A. Fragile brain capillaries that may bleed
    B. Lungs deficient in surfactant, making ventilation difficult
    C. Poor temperature control
    D. Higher likelihood of an infection
    E. All of the above

13. Every delivery should be attended by at least _____ skilled person(s) whose sole responsibility is the management of the newborn.

14. If a high-risk delivery is anticipated, at least _____ skilled person(s), whose sole responsibility is resuscitation and the management of the baby, should be present at the delivery.

15. When a depressed newborn is anticipated at a delivery, resuscitation equipment (should) (should not) be unpacked and ready for use.

16. A baby who was meconium-stained and not vigorous at birth had meconium suctioned from the trachea. She then resumed breathing and became more active. This baby should now receive (routine) (supportive) (ongoing) care.

Birth

APPROXIMATE TIME

30 SECONDS

- Clear of meconium?
- Breathing or crying?
- Good muscle tone?
- Color pink?
- Term gestation?

No

- Provide warmth
- Position; clear airway* (as necessary)
- Dry, stimulate, reposition
- Give O$_2$ (as necessary)

- Evaluate respirations, heart rate, and color

30 SECONDS

30 SECONDS

- Administer epinephrine*

*Endotracheal intubation may be considered at several steps.

Appendix

Neonatal Resuscitation Supplies and Equipment

Suction equipment
Bulb syringe
Mechanical suction and tubing
Suction catheters, 5F or 6F, 8F, 10F or 12F
8F feeding tube and 20-mL syringe
Meconium aspirator

Bag-and-mask equipment
Neonatal resuscitation bag with a pressure-release valve or pressure
    manometer (the bag must be capable of delivering 90% to 100%
    oxygen)
Face masks, newborn and premature sizes (cushioned-rim masks
    preferred)
Oxygen source with flowmeter (flow rate up to 10 L/min) and tubing

Intubation equipment
Laryngoscope with straight blades, No. 0 (preterm) and No. 1 (term)
Extra bulbs and batteries for laryngoscope
Endotracheal tubes, 2.5-, 3.0-, 3.5-, 4.0-mm internal diameter (ID)
Stylet (optional)
Scissors
Tape or securing device for endotracheal tube
Alcohol sponges
CO_2 detector (optional)
Laryngeal mask airway (optional)

Medications
Epinephrine 1:10,000 (0.1 mg/mL) — 3-mL or 10-mL ampules
Isotonic crystalloid (normal saline or Ringer's lactate) for volume
    expansion — 100 or 250 mL
Sodium bicarbonate 4.2% (5mEq/10mL) — 10-mL ampules
Naloxone hydrochloride 0.4 mg/mL — 1-mL ampules, or 1.0 mg/mL
    — 2-mL ampules
Dextrose 10%, 250 mL
Normal saline for flushes
Feeding tube, 5F (optional)
Umbilical vessel catheterization supplies
    Sterile gloves
    Scalpel or scissors
    Povidone-iodine solution
    Umbilical tape
    Umbilical catheters, 3.5F, 5F
    Three-way stopcock
Syringes, 1, 3, 5, 10, 20, 50 mL
Needles, 25, 21, 18 gauge, or puncture device for needleless system

Appendix — *continued*

Neonatal Resuscitation Supplies and Equipment

Miscellaneous
Gloves and appropriate personal protection
Radiant warmer or other heat source
Firm, padded resuscitation surface
Clock (timer optional)
Warmed linens
Stethoscope (neonatal head preferred)
Tape, 1/2 or 3/4 inch
Cardiac monitor and electrodes or pulse oximeter and probe
  (optional for delivery room)
Oropharyngeal airways (0, 00, and 000 sizes or 30-, 40-, and
  50-mm lengths)

Apgar Score

Sign	Score		
	0	1	2
Heart rate	Absent	Slow (<100 beats/min)	≥100 beats/min
Respirations	Absent	Slow, irregular	Good, crying
Muscle tone	Limp	Some flexion	Active motion
Reflex irritability (catheter in nares, tactile stimulation)	No response	Grimace	Cough, sneeze, cry
Color	Blue or pale	Pink body, blue extremities	Completely pink

The Apgar score quantifies and summarizes the response of the newly born infant to the extrauterine environment and to resuscitation. Each of the five signs is awarded a value of 0, 1, or 2. The five values are then added and the sum becomes the Apgar score.

Apgar scores should be assigned at 1 and 5 minutes after birth. When the 5-minute score is less than 7, additional scores should be assigned every 5 minutes for up to 20 minutes. These scores should not be used to dictate appropriate resuscitative actions, nor should interventions for depressed infants be delayed until the 1-minute assessment.

The scores should be recorded in the baby's birth record. Complete documentation of the events taking place during a resuscitation must also include a narrative description of interventions performed and their timing.

Key Points

1. Worldwide, the outcomes of more than 1 million babies per year might be improved through the use of NRP techniques.

2. Most newly born babies are vigorous. Ten percent require some kind of assistance. One percent need major resuscitative measures to survive.

3. Fetal lungs are expanded in utero, but alveoli are fluid filled.

4. The blood vessels in fetal lungs are markedly constricted so that instead of perfusing the lungs, blood is shunted from the pulmonary artery through the ductus arteriosus into the aorta.

5. At birth, the fluid in the alveoli is absorbed into lung tissue and is replaced by air.

6. Exposure to oxygen after birth causes the pulmonary arterioles to relax, permitting a dramatic increase in pulmonary blood flow. The blood absorbs oxygen from the air in the alveoli, and the oxygen-enriched blood is pumped to tissues throughout the baby's body.

7. Lack of oxygen to the newborn's lungs results in sustained constriction of the pulmonary arterioles, preventing systemic arterial blood from becoming oxygenated. Initially, blood flow to the intestines, kidneys, muscles, and skin decreases, while blood flow to the heart and brain is preserved. Continued lack of adequate perfusion and oxygenation can lead to brain damage, damage to other organs, or death.

8. When a fetus/newborn first becomes deprived of oxygen, an initial period of rapid breathing is followed by primary apnea. Primary apnea can be resolved by tactile stimulation.

9. If oxygen deprivation continues, secondary apnea ensues. The heart rate continues to fall, and the blood pressure falls. Secondary apnea cannot be reversed with stimulation; assisted ventilation must be provided.

10. The Apgar score is useful for conveying information about overall status and response to resuscitation. It is not useful for determining the need for resuscitation, what resuscitation steps are necessary, or when to use them.

11. Most, but not all, neonatal resuscitations can be anticipated. It is important to identify the antepartum and intrapartum risk factors that are associated with the need for neonatal resuscitation.

12. Every birth should be attended by at least one person whose primary responsibility is the baby and who is capable of initiating resuscitation. Either that person or someone else who is immediately available should have the skills required to perform a complete resuscitation.

13. When you anticipate a complex resuscitation, recruit additional personnel prior to delivery to be present in the delivery room.

14. Prepare resuscitation equipment prior to the birth.

Key Points — *continued*

15. Protect yourself from exposure to blood and body fluid. Observe standard precautions as defined by hospital policy.

16. Premature babies are at higher risk for needing resuscitation than term babies because
    - Preterm lungs may be deficient in surfactant.
    - Preterm babies are more susceptible to heat loss.
    - Preterm babies are more likely to be born with an infection.
    - Preterm brain vasculature is susceptible to bleeding during stress.

17. All newborns require ongoing observation of breathing, activity, and color. Post-birth care encompasses three levels.
    - Routine care — standard observation
    - Supportive care — frequent evaluation
    - Ongoing care — ongoing evaluation and monitoring in a nursery environment

18. The most important and effective action in neonatal resuscitation is getting oxygen into the baby's lungs.

19. All newborns require initial assessment.
    - Is the amniotic fluid and the baby's skin clear of meconium?
    - Is the newborn breathing or crying?
    - Does the newborn have good muscle tone?
    - Is the newborn pink?
    - Was the baby born at term (37 to 42 weeks' gestation)?

    If any answer is "No," begin resuscitation.

20. Resuscitation occurs over a short period of time.
    - You have approximately 30 seconds to achieve a response from one step before deciding whether you need to go on to the next.
    - Evaluation and decision making are based primarily on respirations, heart rate, and color.

21. The steps of neonatal resuscitation are
    A. Initial steps
       - Provide warmth.
       - Position head and clear airway as necessary.*
       - Dry and stimulate the baby to breathe.
       - Evaluate respirations, heart rate, and color; give oxygen as necessary.
    B. **Provide** positive-pressure ventilation with a resuscitation bag and 100% oxygen.*
    C. **Provide** chest compressions as you continue assisted ventilation.*
    D. **Administer** epinephrine as you continue assisted ventilation and chest compressions.*

    *Consider intubation of the trachea at these points.

Answers to Questions

1. **1** million

2. 10%

3. 1%

4. Chest compressions and medications are **rarely** needed when resuscitating newborns.

5. Before birth, the alveoli are **expanded** and filled with **fluid**.

6. At birth, strong breathing causes **fluid** to be absorbed from the lungs and replaced with **air**.

7. Oxygen causes pulmonary arterioles to **relax**.

8. You should assume **secondary apnea** and you should provide **positive-pressure ventilation**.

9. The baby will be **blue,** his heart rate will **fall**, and his blood pressure will **fall**.

10. A. Apnea or Heart rate **<100 beats per minute**
    B. Provide **positive-pressure ventilation**
    C. Heart rate **<60 beats per minute**
    D. Provide positive-pressure ventilation and **chest compressions**
    E. Heart rate **<60 beats per minute**

11. Resuscitation **should not** be delayed until the 1-minute Apgar score is available.

12. Premature babies have fragile brain capillaries, immature lungs, poor temperature control, and are more likely to have an infection. Therefore, **all of the above** is the correct answer.

13. Every delivery should be attended by at least **one** skilled person.

14. At least **two** skilled persons should be present at a high-risk delivery.

15. Equipment **should** be unpacked if a newborn is anticipated to be depressed at delivery.

16. Since the baby required suctioning of meconium from the airway, she should receive **supportive** care.

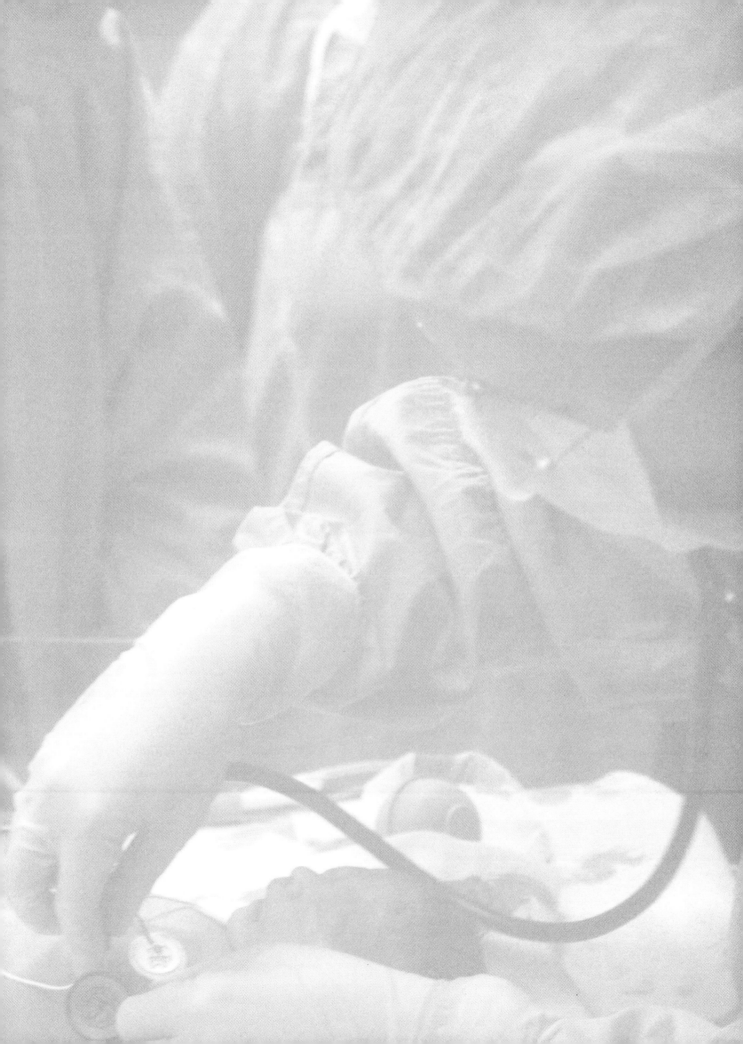

2

Initial Steps
in Resuscitation

In Lesson 2 you will learn how to

- Decide if a newborn needs to be resuscitated.
- Open the airway, and provide the initial steps of resuscitation.
- Resuscitate newborns when meconium is present.
- Provide free-flow oxygen when it is needed.

The following two cases are examples of how the initial steps of evaluation and resuscitation may be used. As you read each case, imagine yourself as part of the resuscitation team. The details of the initial steps will be described in the remainder of the lesson.

Case 1. An uncomplicated delivery

A 24-year-old woman enters the hospital in active labor at term. The membranes ruptured 1 hour before arrival, and the amniotic fluid was clear. The cervix dilates progressively and, after several hours, a baby girl is born vaginally in vertex presentation.

The cord is clamped and cut. Clear secretions are cleaned from the baby's mouth and nose. She immediately breathes spontaneously as she is dried with a warm towel.

She quickly becomes pink, has good muscle tone, and is placed on her mother's chest to remain warm and to complete transition.

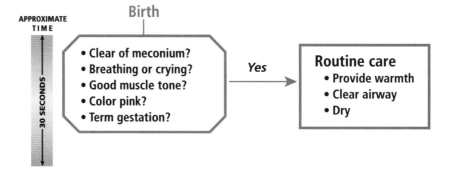

Case 2. Resuscitation involving meconium

A multiparous woman presents at term in early labor. Soon after admission, her membranes rupture, and the fluid is noted to contain thick meconium, similar to "pea soup." Fetal heart rate monitoring shows occasional late decelerations. A judgment is made to allow a vaginal delivery.

After the head is delivered, the nose and mouth are suctioned with a catheter. After the baby is completely born, he has poor tone and minimal respiratory efforts and is cyanotic.

He is placed under a radiant warmer and given free-flow oxygen while his oropharynx is cleared of meconium with a large-bore suction catheter. The trachea is intubated and suction applied to the endotracheal tube as it is being removed from the trachea, but no meconium is recovered. The baby still has weak respiratory efforts and remains cyanotic despite being given 100% free-flow oxygen.

The baby is now dried with a warm towel and stimulated to breathe by flicking the soles of his feet while his head is repositioned to establish his airway. As free-flow oxygen is continued, he immediately begins to breathe more effectively, and the heart rate is measured to be more than 120 bpm.

By 5 minutes after birth, the baby is breathing regularly, has a heart rate of 150 bpm, and remains pink without supplemental oxygen. Several minutes later, he is placed on his mother's chest to complete transition while vital signs and activity are observed closely and monitored frequently for possible deterioration.

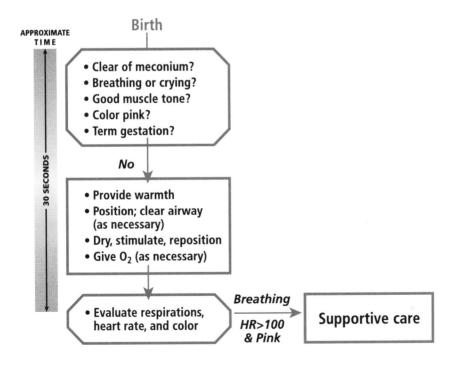

Using the flow diagram and these examples, assume that you are responsible for a baby that has just been delivered.

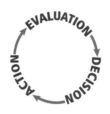

Within a few seconds you have asked yourself the following questions:
• Is the amniotic fluid clear of meconium?
• Is the baby breathing or crying?
• Is there good muscle tone?
• Is the color pink?
• Was the baby born at term?

If the answer to all of these is "Yes," the baby may receive routine care to continue transition. If the answer to any one of these is "No," or the baby was born preterm, the baby will require some form of resuscitation.

The initial steps of resuscitation include the following:
• Providing a warm and dry environment
• Positioning and clearing the airway, particularly if there is meconium present
• Drying and stimulating the baby to breathe while repositioning the head to open the airway
• Giving oxygen, as necessary, to relieve cyanosis

PREMATURITY POINTERS
Preterm babies are more likely to have difficulty with transition and should receive the initial steps of resuscitation as necessary.

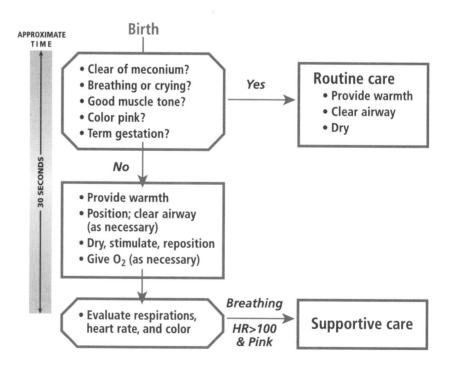

How do you determine whether the baby requires resuscitation?

• *Is the baby clear of meconium?*
This is a very important question. If meconium is present in the amniotic fluid or on the baby's skin and the baby is not vigorous, you should intubate and suction the trachea before performing the other resuscitation steps. No more than a few seconds should elapse while you make this determination.

• *Is the baby breathing or crying?*
Breathing will be evident by watching the baby's chest. A vigorous cry also indicates breathing. However, don't be misled by a baby who is gasping. Gasping is a series of deep single or stacked inspirations that occur in the presence of hypoxia and/or ischemia. It is indicative of severe neurologic and respiratory depression.

 A gasp usually indicates a severe problem and requires the same intervention as no respiratory efforts at all (apnea).

• *Is there good muscle tone?*
Healthy term babies should have flexed extremities and be active.

• *Is the baby pink?*
A baby's skin color, changing from blue to pink in the first several seconds following delivery, can provide the most rapid and visible indicator of adequate breathing and circulation. The baby's skin color is best determined by looking at the central part of the body. Cyanosis caused by too little oxygen in the blood will appear as a blue hue to the lips, tongue, and central trunk. Healthy newborns sometimes will have central cyanosis, which should then become pink within a few seconds after birth. "Acrocyanosis," which is a blue hue to only the hands and feet, may persist longer. Acrocyanosis without central cyanosis does not generally indicate that the baby's blood oxygen level is low. Only central cyanosis requires intervention. Turn to Center Page A to see color pictures of central cyanosis versus acrocyanosis (Figures A-2 and A-4).

• Clear of meconium?
• Breathing or crying?
• Good muscle tone?
• Color pink?

See page A in the center of the book for color photographs of central cyanosis and acrocyanosis.

> **Initial Steps**
> • Provide warmth
> • Position; clear airway
>   (as necessary)
> • Dry, stimulate,
>   reposition
> • Give O$_2$ (as necessary)

What are the initial steps and how are they administered?

If the baby is term and vigorous, the initial steps may be provided in modified form, as described in Lesson 1 (page 1-15 under "Routine Care"). Babies born preterm are more likely to have difficulty with transition and should be carefully evaluated, usually under a radiant warmer, while the initial steps are being performed.

Once you have decided that resuscitation is required, all of the initial steps should be initiated within a few seconds. Although they are listed as "initial" and are given in a particular order, they should continue to be applied throughout the resuscitation process.

• *Provide warmth*
The baby should be placed under a radiant warmer, where the resuscitation team will have easy access to the baby and the radiant heat will help to reduce heat loss (Figure 2.1). The baby should not be covered with blankets or towels. Leave the baby uncovered to allow full visualization and to permit the radiant heat to reach the baby.

PREMATURITY POINTERS
Premature babies are particularly vulnerable to cold stress. Their larger surface-area-to-body-mass ratio, thin permeable skin, decreased amount of subcutaneous fat, and diminished metabolic response to cold result in rapid heat loss and decrease in body temperature. Babies born prematurely should have all steps taken to reduce heat loss, even if they do not initially appear to require resuscitation.

• *Position by slightly extending the neck*
The baby should be **positioned** on the back or side, with the neck slightly extended in the "sniffing" position. This will bring the posterior pharynx, larynx, and trachea in line, which will facilitate unrestricted air entry. This alignment is also best to assist ventilation with bag and mask and/or to place an endotracheal tube.

Care should be taken to prevent hyperextension or flexion of the neck, since either may restrict air entry (Figure 2.2).

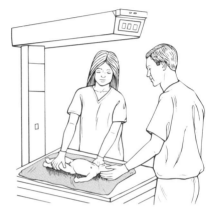

Figure 2.1. Radiant warmer for resuscitating newborns

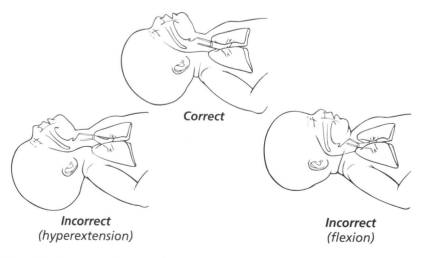

Correct

*Incorrect
(hyperextension)*

*Incorrect
(flexion)*

Figure 2.2. Correct and incorrect head positions for resuscitation

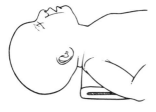

To help maintain the correct position, you may place a rolled blanket or towel under the shoulders (Figure 2.3). This shoulder roll may be particularly useful if the baby has a large occiput resulting from molding, edema, or prematurity.

• *Clear airway*
If meconium was present in the amniotic fluid, the person delivering the baby should have suctioned the oropharynx and nares with a catheter or bulb syringe before delivering the shoulders.

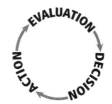

After delivery, the appropriate method for clearing the airway further will depend on the
(1) Presence of meconium
(2) Baby's level of activity

Figure 2.3. Optional shoulder roll for maintaining correct head position

Study the flow diagram below to understand how you suction newborns with meconium.

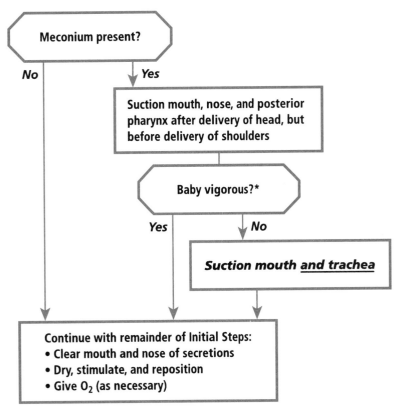

*"Vigorous" is defined as strong respiratory efforts, good muscle tone, and a heart rate greater than 100 bpm. The technique of determining the heart rate is described at the end of this lesson.

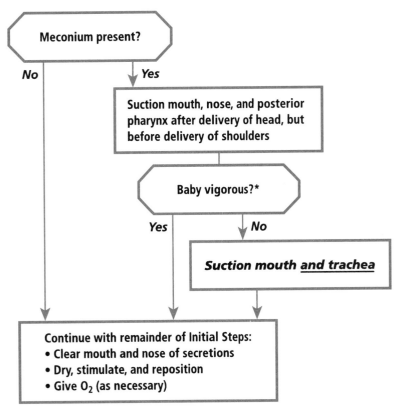

What do you do if meconium is present and the baby is *not* vigorous?

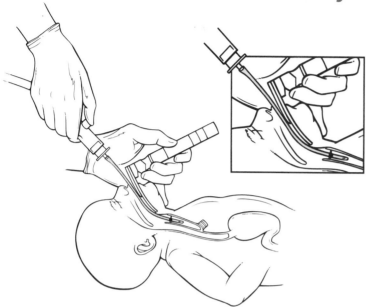

Figure 2.4. Visualizing the glottis and suctioning meconium from the trachea using a laryngoscope and endotracheal tube (see Lesson 5 for details)

If the baby has depressed respirations, depressed muscle tone, and/or a heart rate less than 100 bpm, direct suctioning of the trachea soon after delivery is indicated before many respirations have occurred. The following steps can reduce the chances of the baby developing meconium aspiration syndrome — a very serious respiratory disorder:

* Administer free-flow oxygen throughout the suctioning procedure.

* Insert a laryngoscope and use a 12F or 14F suction catheter to clear the mouth and posterior pharynx so that you can visualize the glottis (Figure 2.4).

* Insert an endotracheal tube into the trachea.

* Attach the endotracheal tube to a suction source. (A special aspirator device will be needed.) (Figure 2.4)

* Apply suction as the tube is slowly withdrawn.

* Repeat as necessary until little additional meconium is recovered, or until the baby's heart rate indicates that resuscitation must proceed without delay.

Details of performing endotracheal intubation and suctioning are described in Lesson 5. Individuals who will be initiating resuscitation, but who will not be intubating newborns, should still be competent in assisting with endotracheal intubation. This also is described in Lesson 5.

Note: Some previous recommendations have suggested that endotracheal suctioning should be determined by whether the meconium has "thick," versus "thin," consistency. While it may be reasonable to speculate that thick meconium might be more hazardous than thin, there are currently no clinical studies that warrant basing suctioning guidelines on meconium consistency.

Also, various techniques such as squeezing the chest, inserting a finger in the baby's mouth, or externally occluding the airway have been proposed to prevent babies from aspirating meconium. None of these techniques have been subjected to rigorous research evaluation and all may be harmful to the baby. They are not recommended.

What do you do if meconium is present and the baby *is* vigorous?

If the baby has a normal respiratory effort, normal muscle tone, and a heart rate greater than 100 bpm, simply use a bulb syringe or large-bore suction catheter (12F or 14F) to clear secretions and any meconium from the mouth and nose. This procedure is described in the next section.

 Check yourself!

(The answers are in the preceding section and at the end of the lesson.)

1. A newborn who is breathing well, has pink color, and has no meconium in the amniotic fluid or on the skin (does) (does not) need resuscitation.

2. A newborn with meconium who is not vigorous (will) (will not) need to have a laryngoscope inserted and be suctioned with an endotracheal tube.

3. When deciding which babies need tracheal suctioning, the term "vigorous" is defined by what three characteristics?
   (1)_____
   (2)_____
   (3)_____

4. When a suction catheter is used to clear the oropharynx of meconium before inserting an endotracheal tube, the appropriate size is _____F or_____F

How do you clear the airway if no meconium is present?

Secretions may be removed from the airway by wiping the nose and mouth with a towel or by suctioning with a bulb syringe or suction catheter. If the newborn has copious secretions coming from the mouth, turn the head to the side. This will allow secretions to collect in the cheek where they can be removed easily.

Use a bulb syringe or a catheter attached to mechanical suction to remove fluid that appears to be blocking the airway. When using suction from the wall or from a pump, the suction pressure should be set so that when the suction tubing is blocked, the negative pressure (vacuum) reads approximately 100 mm Hg.

The mouth is suctioned before the nose to ensure that there is nothing for the newborn to aspirate if he or she should gasp when the nose is suctioned. You can remember "mouth before nose" by thinking "M" comes before "N" in the alphabet (Figure 2.5). If material in the mouth and nose is not removed before the newborn breathes, the material can be aspirated into the trachea and lungs. When this occurs, the respiratory consequences can be serious.

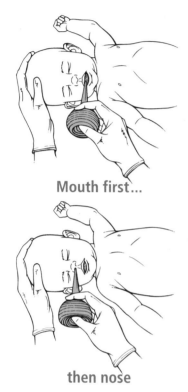

Mouth first...

then nose

Figure 2.5. Suctioning the mouth and nose; "M" before "N"

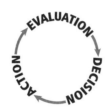

Caution: When you suction, particularly when using a catheter, be careful not to suction vigorously or deeply. Stimulation of the posterior pharynx during the first few minutes after birth can produce a vagal response, causing severe bradycardia or apnea. Brief, gentle suctioning with a bulb syringe is usually adequate to remove secretions.

If bradycardia occurs during suctioning, stop suctioning and re-evaluate the heart rate.

Suctioning, in addition to clearing the airway to allow unrestricted air entry to the lungs, also provides a degree of *stimulation*. In some cases this is all the stimulation needed to initiate respirations in the newborn.

Once the airway is clear, what should be done to stimulate breathing and further prevent heat loss?

• *Dry, stimulate to breathe, and reposition*

Often, positioning the baby and suctioning secretions will provide enough stimulation to initiate breathing. Drying will also provide stimulation. Drying the body and head will also help to prevent heat loss. If two people are present, the second person can be drying the baby while the first person is positioning and clearing the airway.

As part of preparation for a resuscitation, you should have several pre-warmed absorbent towels or blankets available. The baby initially can be placed on one of these towels, which can be used to dry most of the fluid. This towel should then be discarded, and fresh pre-warmed towels or blankets should be used for continued drying and stimulation.

While you dry the baby, and thereafter, be sure to keep the head in the "sniffing" position to maintain a good airway (Figure 2.6).

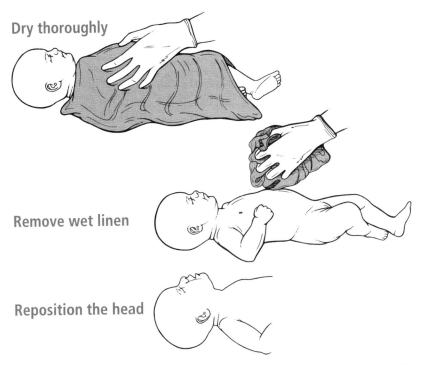

Dry thoroughly

Remove wet linen

Reposition the head

Figure 2.6. Drying and removing wet linen to prevent heat loss and repositioning the head to ensure an open airway

What other forms of stimulation may help a baby breathe?

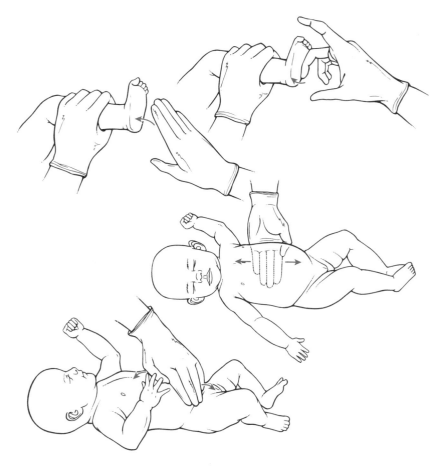

Both drying and suctioning stimulate the newborn. For many newborns, these steps are enough to induce respirations. If the newborn does not have adequate respirations, additional tactile stimulation may be provided *briefly* to stimulate breathing.

It is important for you to understand the correct methods of tactile stimulation. Even if you do not use them at this point in a resuscitation, you may use them later, after you have initiated respirations with bag-and-mask ventilation, to stimulate the newborn to continue breathing.

Safe and appropriate methods of providing additional tactile stimulation include

- Slapping or flicking the soles of the feet

- Gently rubbing the newborn's back, trunk, or extremities (Figure 2.7)

Figure 2.7. Acceptable methods of stimulating a baby to breathe

 Overly vigorous stimulation is not helpful and can cause serious injury. *Do not* shake the baby.

Remember, if a newborn is in primary apnea, almost any form of stimulation will initiate breathing. If a baby is in secondary apnea, no amount of stimulation will work. Therefore, one or two slaps or flicks to the soles of the feet, or rubbing the back once or twice, should be sufficient. If the newborn remains apneic, positive-pressure ventilation should be initiated immediately, as described in Lesson 3.

 Continued use of tactile stimulation in a newborn who is not breathing wastes valuable time. For persistent apnea, give positive-pressure ventilation.

What forms of stimulation may be hazardous?

Certain actions that were used in the past to provide tactile stimulation to apneic newborns can harm a baby and should not be used.

Harmful Actions	Potential Consequences
Slapping the back	Bruising
Squeezing the rib cage	Fractures, pneumothorax, respiratory distress, death
Forcing thighs onto abdomen	Rupture of liver or spleen
Dilating anal sphincter	Tearing of anal sphincter
Using hot or cold compresses or baths	Hyperthermia, hypothermia, burns
Shaking	Brain damage

PREMATURITY POINTERS

Premature babies have a very fragile portion of their brains called the germinal matrix. This structure consists of a network of capillaries that are prone to rupture if the baby is handled too vigorously or if the head is aggressively placed in a very dependent position (Trendelenburg's position). A ruptured germinal matrix results in intracranial hemorrhage that can be associated with lifelong disability. Therefore, if premature babies require resuscitation, particular care should be taken not to stimulate them too vigorously. Premature babies also are more likely to require positive-pressure ventilation, as described in Lesson 3.

Check yourself!

(The answers are in the preceding section and at the end of the lesson.)

5. Which drawing shows the correct way to position a newborn's head for suctioning?

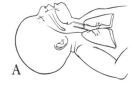 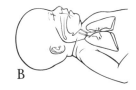 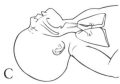

A   B   C

6. In suctioning a baby's nose and mouth, the rule is to first suction the _____ and then the _____.

7. Write a check mark next to the correct ways to stimulate a newborn.
    ____ Slap on the back   ____ Slap on the sole of foot   ____ Rub the back   ____ Squeeze the rib cage

8. If a baby is in secondary apnea, stimulation alone (will) (will not) stimulate breathing.

9. A newborn is still not breathing after stimulation. The next action should be to administer
    ____ Additional stimulation   ____ Positive-pressure ventilation

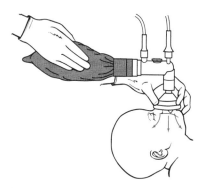

Figure 2.8. Using a flow-inflating bag to deliver free-flow oxygen. Hold the mask close to the face, but not so tight that pressure builds up.

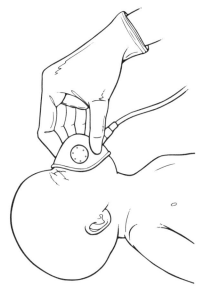

Figure 2.9. Oxygen mask held close to the baby's face to give close to 100% oxygen

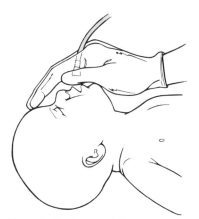

Figure 2.10. Oxygen delivered by tubing held in cupped hand over baby's face

What do you do if the baby is breathing, but there is central cyanosis?

• *Give free-flow oxygen*

Most babies will have begun to breathe and will have established regular respirations after suctioning of the airway, drying, and stimulation. However, some of these babies will still have central cyanosis. In these circumstances, free-flow 100% oxygen should be given. Deprivation of oxygen to vital tissues is one of the primary reasons for the clinical consequences associated with perinatal compromise.

Free-flow oxygen refers to blowing oxygen over the baby's nose so that the baby breathes oxygen-enriched air. For a brief time, this can be accomplished by using one of the following delivery methods:

• *Flow*-inflating bag and mask

• Oxygen tubing

• Oxygen mask

! Free-flow oxygen cannot be given reliably by a mask attached to a *self*-inflating bag. (See Lesson 3.)

When a baby is cyanotic during resuscitation, it is important to deliver as close to 100% oxygen as possible without allowing it to mix with room air. Your wall or portable oxygen source sends 100% oxygen through the tubing. As oxygen flows out of the tubing or mask, it mixes with room air, which contains only 21% oxygen. The concentration of oxygen that reaches the baby's nose is determined by the amount of 100% oxygen coming from the tube or mask (usually at least 5 L/min) and the amount of room air it must pass through to reach the baby. Therefore, it is important to have the oxygen mask or tube very close to the baby's nose to deliver the highest possible concentration of oxygen (Figure 2.8).

The highest concentration of free-flow oxygen is achieved most reliably with an oxygen mask or a flow-inflating resuscitation bag and mask, which you will learn about in Lesson 3. In either case, the mask should be held close to the face to keep the concentration of oxygen as high as possible, but not so tight that pressure builds up within the mask (Figure 2.9).

If a mask is not immediately available, try to keep the oxygen concentrated around the baby's airway by using a funnel or by cupping your hand around the baby's face and the oxygen tubing (Figure 2.10).

How much oxygen should be given, and does it need to be heated?

You should provide enough oxygen for the newborn to become pink. After the resuscitation, once respirations and heart rate are stable and you have established that the newborn requires ongoing supplemental oxygen, pulse oximetry and arterial blood gas determinations should guide the appropriate oxygen concentration.

When oxygen comes from a compressed source in the wall or from a tank, it is very cold and dry. To prevent heat loss and drying of the respiratory mucosa, oxygen given to newborns for long periods should be heated and humidified. However, during resuscitation, dry unheated oxygen may be given for the few minutes required to stabilize the newborn's condition.

Avoid giving unheated and unhumidified oxygen at high flow rates (above approximately 10 L/min), because convective heat loss can become a significant problem. A flow rate of 5 L/min is usually adequate for free-flow oxygen during a resuscitation.

How do you know when to stop giving oxygen?

Once the newborn becomes pink, the supplemental oxygen should be *gradually* withdrawn until the newborn can remain pink while breathing room air.

Newborns who become cyanotic as supplemental oxygen is withdrawn should continue to receive enough oxygen to remain pink until arterial blood gas determinations and oximetry can be used to adjust oxygen levels to the normal range.

If cyanosis persists despite 100% free-flow oxygen, a trial of positive-pressure ventilation may be indicated (see Lesson 3), and/or a diagnosis of cyanotic congenital heart disease should be considered (see Lesson 7).

Check yourself!

(The answers are in the preceding section and at the end of the lesson.)

10. A newborn is breathing and is cyanotic. Your initial steps are to *(Check all that are appropriate.)*

    ____ Place him on a radiant warmer.

    ____ Suction his mouth and nose.

    ____ Dry and stimulate.

    ____ Remove all wet linen.

    ____ Give him free-flow oxygen.

11. A newborn is covered with meconium, is breathing well, has normal muscle tone, has a heart rate of 120 beats per minute, and is pink. The correct action is to

    ____ Insert a laryngoscope and suction his trachea with an endotracheal tube.

    ____ Suction the mouth and nose with a bulb syringe or suction catheter.

12. Which drawings show the correct way to give free-flow oxygen to a baby who is cyanotic but is breathing well?

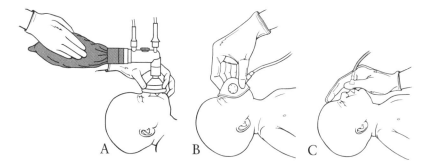

A   B   C

Now that you have warmed, positioned, cleared the airway, dried, stimulated, and given oxygen as necessary, what do you do next?

Evaluate the baby

Your next step is to evaluate the newborn to determine if further resuscitation actions are indicated. The vital signs that you evaluate are as follows:

• *Respirations*

There should be good chest rise, and the rate and depth of respirations should increase after a few seconds of tactile stimulation. Remember, gasping respirations are ineffective and require the same intervention as for apnea.

• *Heart rate*

The heart rate should be more than 100 bpm. The easiest and quickest method of determining the heart rate is to feel for a pulse at the base of the umbilical cord, where it attaches to the baby's abdomen (Figure 2.11). However, sometimes the umbilical vessels are constricted so that the pulse is not palpable. Therefore, if you cannot feel a pulse, you should listen for the heartbeat over the left side of the chest using a stethoscope. If you can feel a pulse or hear the heartbeat, tap it out on the bed so that others will also know the heart rate.

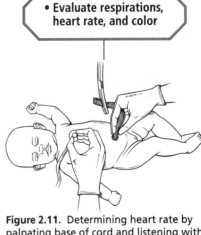

• Evaluate respirations, heart rate, and color

Figure 2.11. Determining heart rate by palpating base of cord and listening with a stethoscope

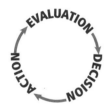

Counting the number of beats in 6 seconds and multiplying by 10 can provide a quick estimate of the beats per minute.

• *Color*

The baby should have pink lips and a pink trunk. Once adequate heart rate and ventilation are established, there should not be *central cyanosis,* which indicates hypoxemia.

What do you do if any of these vital signs (respirations, heart rate, or color) are abnormal?

 The most effective and important action in resuscitating a compromised newborn is to assist ventilation.

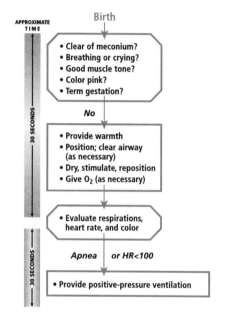

No matter which vital sign is abnormal, almost all compromised newborns will respond to establishment or improvement of ventilation. Therefore, after you have taken a few seconds to minimize heat loss, clear the airway, and try to stimulate spontaneous respirations, the next appropriate action should be to assist ventilation. This will be accomplished by providing positive pressure to the airway with a bag and mask, as described in Lesson 3.

Remember, the entire process to this point should take no more than 30 seconds (or perhaps a bit longer if suctioning of meconium from the trachea was required).

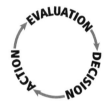 Administering free-flow oxygen or continuing to provide tactile stimulation to a nonbreathing newborn or to a newborn whose heart rate is less than 100 bpm is of little or no value and only delays appropriate treatment.

Lesson 2 Review

(The answers are at the end of the lesson.)

1. A newborn who is breathing well, has pink color, and has no meconium in the amniotic fluid or on the skin (does) (does not) need resuscitation.

2. A newborn with meconium who is not vigorous (will) (will not) need to have a laryngoscope inserted and be suctioned with an endotracheal tube.

3. When deciding which babies need tracheal suctioning, the term "vigorous" is defined by what three characteristics?
   (1)_____
   (2)_____
   (3)_____

4. When a suction catheter is used to clear the oropharynx of meconium before inserting an endotracheal tube, the appropriate size is _____F or_____F.

5. Which drawing shows the correct way to position a newborn's head for suctioning?

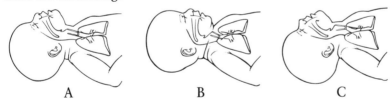

   A   B   C

6. In suctioning a baby's nose and mouth, the rule is to first suction the _____and then the _____.

7. Write a check mark next to the correct ways to stimulate a newborn.
   ____Slap on the back   ____Slap on the sole of foot
   ____Rub the back   ____Squeeze the rib cage

8. If a baby is in secondary apnea, stimulation alone (will) (will not) stimulate breathing.

9. A newborn is still not breathing after stimulation.
   The next action should be to administer
   ____Additional stimulation   ____Positive-pressure ventilation

Lesson 2 Review — *continued*

(The answers are at the end of the lesson.)

10. A newborn is breathing and is cyanotic. Your initial steps are to *(Check all that are appropriate.)*
    ___Place him on a radiant warmer.   ___Remove all wet linen.
    ___Suction his mouth and nose.   ___Give him free-flow oxygen.
    ___Dry and stimulate.

11. A newborn is covered with meconium, is breathing well, has normal muscle tone, has a heart rate of 120 beats per minute, and is pink. The correct action is to
    ___Insert a laryngoscope and suction his trachea with an endotracheal tube.
    ___Suction the mouth and nose with a bulb syringe or suction catheter.

12. Which drawings show the correct way to give free-flow oxygen to a baby who is cyanotic but is breathing well?

13. If you need to give oxygen for longer than a few minutes, the oxygen should be _____ and _____.

14. You have stimulated a newborn, suctioned her mouth, and given her free-flow oxygen. It is now 30 seconds after birth, and she is still not breathing and is pale. Her heart rate is 80 beats per minute. Your next action should be to
    ___Continue stimulation and free-flow oxygen.
    ___Provide positive-pressure ventilation with 100% oxygen by bag and mask.

15. You count a newborn's heartbeats for 6 seconds and count 6 beats. You would report the heart rate as _____.

Performance Checklist
Lesson 2 — Initial Steps in Resuscitation

Instructor: The participant should be instructed to talk through the procedure as it is demonstrated. Judge the performance of each step and check (✓) the box when the action is completed correctly. If done incorrectly, circle the box so that you can discuss that step later. You will need to provide information at several points concerning the condition of the baby.

Learner: To successfully complete this checklist, you should be able to perform all the steps and make all the correct decisions in the procedure. You should talk through the procedure as you perform it.

Equipment and Supplies

Newborn resuscitation manikin

Radiant warmer or table to
   simulate warmer

Gloves (or may simulate this)

Bulb syringe or suction catheter

Stethoscope

Shoulder roll

Blanket or towel to dry newborn

Self-inflating bag
   or

Flow-inflating bag with
   pressure manometer and
   oxygen source

Flowmeter
   (or may simulate this)

Masks (term and preterm sizes)

Method to administer
   free-flow oxygen (oxygen
   mask, oxygen tubing, or
   flow-inflating bag and mask)

Laryngoscope and blade

Suction catheter

Endotracheal tube

Meconium aspirator

Clock with second hand

Mechanical suction and tubing
   (or may simulate this)

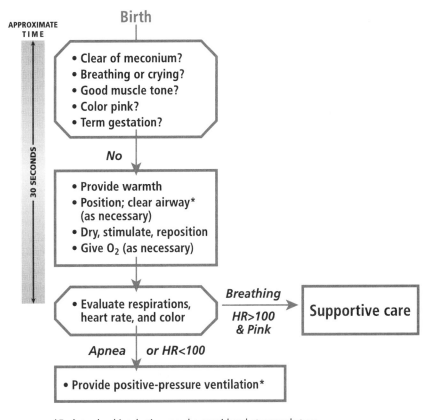

*Endotracheal intubation may be considered at several steps.

Performance Checklist
Lesson 2 — Initial Steps in Resuscitation

Name _____ Instructor _____ Date _____

Instructor's questions are in quotes. Learner's questions and correct responses are in bold type. Instructor should check boxes as the learner answers correctly.

"A newborn has just been delivered. Demonstrate how you would evaluate and care for this newborn. You may ask me any questions you would like to know about the newborn's condition as you progress."

☐ **Learner assesses if there was meconium in the amniotic fluid or on the baby's skin.**

"Yes, meconium is present."   "No, there is no meconium."

☐ **Assesses if the baby is vigorous**
- **Is there good respiratory effort?**
- **Is there good muscle tone?**
- **Is the heart rate >100 bpm?**

"No." (to any question)   "Yes." (to all questions)

☐ **Indicates that tracheal suctioning would be required**

☐ **Assesses remaining items of evaluation block**
- **Is the baby breathing or crying?**
- **Is there good muscle tone?**
- **Is the baby pink?**
- **Was the baby born at term?**

"No." (to any question)   "Yes." (to all questions)

☐ **Indicates that baby will require the initial steps**

☐ **Indicates that baby can receive routine care**
- **Keeping baby warm**
- **Ensuring clear airway**
- **Observing vital signs**

Initial Steps

☐ Places baby on preheated radiant warmer (unless already there following tracheal suctioning)

☐ Positions baby with neck slightly extended

☐ Suctions mouth, then nose

☐ Dries amniotic fluid from body and head and stimulates baby to breathe

☐ Removes wet linen from contact with baby

☐ Repositions baby with neck slightly extended

☐ Administers oxygen as necessary

☐ Evaluates respirations, heart rate, and color

"Breathing"
"Heart rate is above 100 bpm"
"Pink or acrocyanosis"

"Breathing"
"Heart rate is above 100 bpm"
"Central cyanosis"

"Apnea" or "Gasping respirations" or "Heart rate is below 100 bpm"

☐ **Provides free-flow oxygen, 90% to 100%**

☐ **Evaluates color**

"Pink"

"Cyanotic"

☐ **Slowly withdraws oxygen, keeping baby pink**

☐ **Indicates need for positive-pressure ventilation with 90% to 100% oxygen**

☐ **Continues to observe if heart rate, respirations, and color normal**

☐ **Completes Initial Assessment, Initial Steps, and Evaluation in approximately 30 seconds**

Rev 11/01

Key Points

1. Initial assessment, performed within a few seconds, determines if routine care is indicated or if some degree of resuscitation is required. The five questions to ask are

   • Is the amniotic fluid clear of meconium?

   • Is the baby breathing or crying?

   • Is there good muscle tone?

   • Is the color pink?

   • Was the baby born at term?

   If the answer is "No" to any of these questions, begin resuscitation.

2. All newborns with meconium in the amniotic fluid should have the meconium suctioned from the pharynx before delivery of the shoulders.

3. If meconium is present and the newborn is *not* vigorous, suction the baby's trachea before proceeding with any other steps. If the newborn *is* vigorous, suction the mouth and nose only, and proceed with resuscitation as required.

4. "Vigorous" is defined as a newborn who has strong respiratory efforts, good muscle tone, and a heart rate greater than 100 beats per minute.

5. Open the airway by positioning the newborn in a "sniffing" position.

6. Suction the newborn's mouth before his nose.

7. Appropriate forms of tactile stimulation are

   • Slapping or flicking the soles of the feet

   • Gently rubbing the back

8. Continued use of tactile stimulation in an apneic newborn wastes valuable time. For persistent apnea, begin positive-pressure ventilation promptly.

9. Free-flow oxygen is indicated for central cyanosis. Acceptable methods for administering free-flow oxygen are

   • Oxygen mask held firmly over the baby's face

   • Oxygen tubing cupped closely over the baby's mouth and nose

   • Mask from the flow-inflating bag held closely over the baby's mouth and nose

10. Free-flow oxygen cannot be given reliably by a mask attached to a self-inflating bag.

11. Decisions and actions during newborn resuscitation are based on the newborn's

    • Respirations • Heart rate • Color

12. Determine a newborn's heart rate by counting how many beats are in 6 seconds, then multiplying by 10. For example, if you count 8 beats in 6 seconds, announce the baby's heart rate as 80 beats per minute.

Answers to Questions

1. **Does not** need resuscitation.

2. **Will** need to have a laryngoscope inserted and be suctioned.

3. "Vigorous" is defined as: **(1) strong respiratory efforts, (2) good muscle tone, and (3) heart rate greater than 100 beats per minute.**

4. A **12F or 14F** suction catheter should be used to suction meconium.

5. Correct head position is **A:**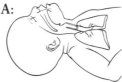

6. First suction the **mouth** and then the **nose**.

7. Stimulate by **slapping the sole of the foot** and/or **rubbing the back**.

8. Stimulation alone **will not** stimulate breathing if the baby is in secondary apnea.

9. If not breathing after stimulation, **provide positive-pressure ventilation**.

10. **All actions are indicated.**

11. Since the newborn is active, he does not need to have his trachea suctioned, but you should **suction the mouth and nose with a bulb syringe or suction catheter**.

12. **All drawings are correct.**

13. The oxygen should be **warmed** and **humidified**.

14. She should receive **positive-pressure ventilation with 100% oxygen by bag and mask**.

15. If you count 6 heartbeats in 6 seconds, report the baby's heart rate as **60 beats per minute** (6 x 10 = 60).

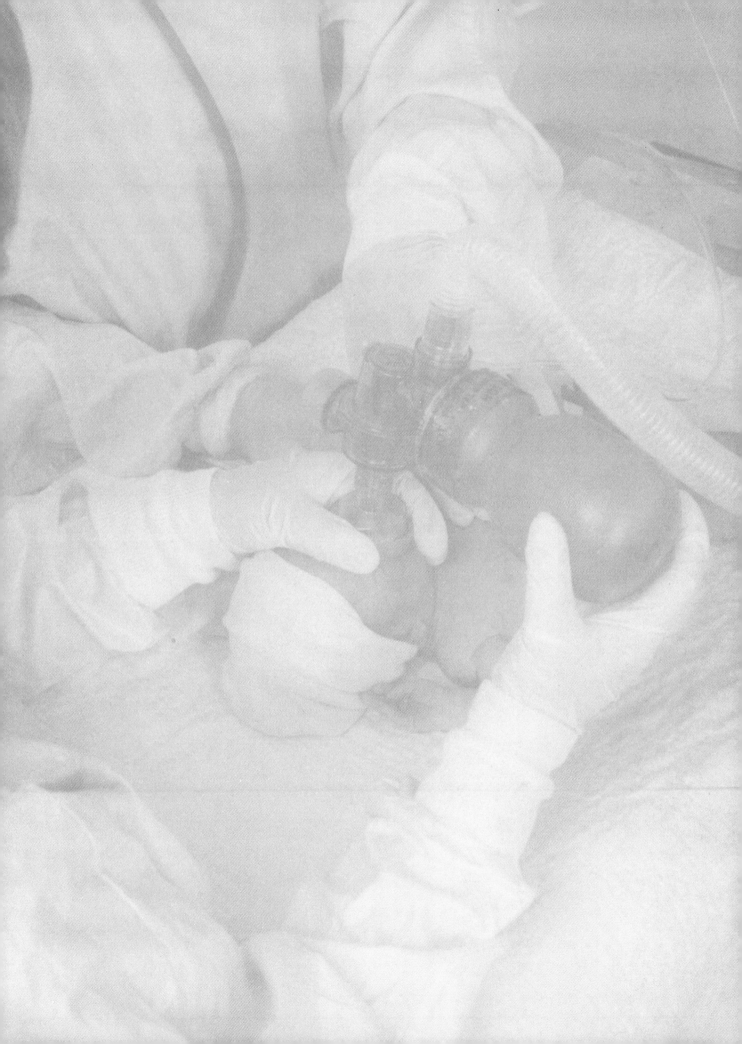

Use of a Resuscitation Bag and Mask

In Lesson 3 you will learn

- When to give bag-and-mask ventilation
- The differences between *flow-inflating* and *self-inflating* bags
- The operation of each type of bag
- The correct placement of masks on the newborn's face
- Testing and troubleshooting each type of bag
- Evaluating the success of bag-and-mask ventilation

The following case is an example of how a bag and mask can be used to provide positive-pressure ventilation during resuscitation. As you read the case, imagine yourself as part of the resuscitation team. The details of this step will then be described in the remainder of the lesson.

Case 3. Resuscitation with bag and mask and 100% oxygen

A 20-year-old woman with pregnancy-induced hypertension has labor induced at 37 weeks' gestation. Several late decelerations of fetal heart rate are noted, but labor progresses quickly, and a baby girl is delivered rapidly.

She is taken to the radiant warmer, where the resuscitation team finds her to be apneic, limp, and cyanotic.

She is appropriately positioned to open her airway, while her mouth and nose are cleared of secretions with a bulb syringe. She is dried with warmed towels, wet linen is removed, her head is repositioned, and further attempts to stimulate her to breathe are provided by flicking the soles of her feet.

No spontaneous respirations are noted after these stimulation activities. She is then given positive-pressure ventilation with a bag and mask, using 100% oxygen.

After 30 seconds of assisted ventilation, her heart rate is checked and found to be 120 beats per minute (bpm) and, after another 30 seconds, she begins to breathe spontaneously. Assisted ventilation is gradually discontinued and she is given free-flow oxygen as further stimulation is provided by gentle rubbing of her extremities. The supplemental oxygen is then gradually withdrawn.

Several minutes after birth, the baby is breathing regularly, has a heart rate of 150 bpm, and remains pink without supplemental oxygen. After a few more minutes of observation, she is moved to the nursery for ongoing care, where vital signs and activity can be monitored closely for deterioration.

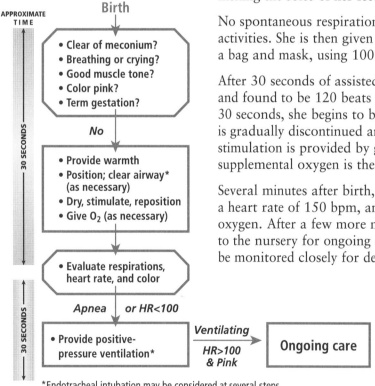

APPROXIMATE TIME

Birth

- Clear of meconium?
- Breathing or crying?
- Good muscle tone?
- Color pink?
- Term gestation?

No

30 SECONDS

- Provide warmth
- Position; clear airway* (as necessary)
- Dry, stimulate, reposition
- Give O₂ (as necessary)

- Evaluate respirations, heart rate, and color

Apnea | *or HR<100*

30 SECONDS

- Provide positive-pressure ventilation*

Ventilating
HR>100 & Pink

Ongoing care

*Endotracheal intubation may be considered at several steps.

What will this lesson cover?

In this lesson you will learn how to prepare and use a resuscitation bag and mask to deliver positive-pressure ventilation.

You learned in Lesson 2 how to determine within a few seconds whether some form of resuscitation will be required and how to take the initial steps of resuscitation.

You start resuscitation by minimizing heat loss; positioning; clearing the airway; stimulating the baby to breathe by drying as you reposition the head; and assessing respirations, heart rate, and color. If the baby is breathing but is cyanotic, you administer 100% free-flow oxygen.

If the baby still is not breathing or is gasping, the heart rate is less than 100 bpm, and/or the color remains cyanotic despite 100% oxygen, the next step is to provide positive-pressure ventilation with a bag and mask.

Ventilation of the lungs is the single most important and most effective step in cardiopulmonary resuscitation of the compromised newly born baby.

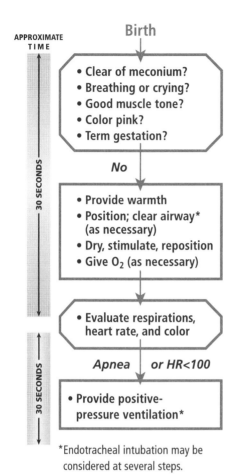

APPROXIMATE TIME

Birth

- Clear of meconium?
- Breathing or crying?
- Good muscle tone?
- Color pink?
- Term gestation?

No

30 SECONDS

- Provide warmth
- Position; clear airway* (as necessary)
- Dry, stimulate, reposition
- Give O_2 (as necessary)

- Evaluate respirations, heart rate, and color

Apnea | *or HR<100*

30 SECONDS

- Provide positive-pressure ventilation*

*Endotracheal intubation may be considered at several steps.

What are the different types of resuscitation bags available to ventilate newborns?

There are two types of resuscitation bags, and they work in quite different ways.

1. The *flow-inflating bag* (also called an anesthesia bag) fills only when oxygen from a compressed source flows into it.

2. The *self-inflating bag* fills spontaneously after it is squeezed, pulling oxygen or air into the bag.

The flow-inflating bag is collapsed when not in use, and it looks like a deflated balloon (Figure 3.1). It inflates only when oxygen is forced into the bag and the opening of the bag is sealed, as when the mask is placed tightly on a baby's face. Its inflation and function are dependent on a compressed gas source.

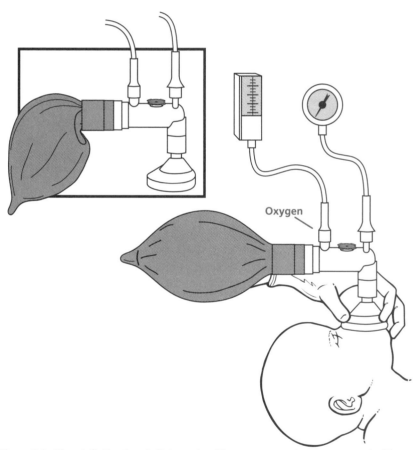

Oxygen

Figure 3.1. Flow-inflating bag inflates only with a compressed gas source and with mask sealed on face; otherwise, the bag remains deflated (inset).

The self-inflating bag, as its name implies, inflates automatically without a compressed gas source (Figure 3.2). It remains inflated at all times and does not depend on a compressed gas source for inflation.

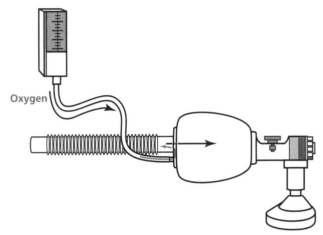

Figure 3.2. Self-inflating bag remains inflated without gas flow and without mask sealed on face. However, it is shown with an oxygen line attached since oxygen is recommended during neonatal resuscitation.

In the next two sections you will learn the general characteristics of both types of bags. In subsequent sections you will learn the details of the type of bag that is used in your hospital.

What are the advantages and disadvantages of each type of bag?

The flow-inflating bag (Figure 3.3) requires a compressed gas source for inflation. When the gas (100% oxygen) flows into the bag, it will continue through the patient outlet without inflating the bag. To make the bag inflate, you need to keep the gas from escaping by having the face mask sealed tightly against the newborn's face. Therefore, when a newborn is being resuscitated, the bag will not fill unless there is gas flow and the mask is tightly sealed over the baby's mouth and nose.

Having a good seal between the mask and the baby's face is important for both types of bags, as a tight seal is necessary to achieve sufficient positive pressure to inflate the baby's lungs. Therefore, this "disadvantage" of requiring a tight seal for the bag to inflate is also an advantage, in that you can quickly tell if there is not a tight seal.

Flow-inflating bags are also generally more sensitive than self-inflating bags. With experience you will be able to judge the relative stiffness of the baby's lungs as you squeeze the bag.

Finally, since flow-inflating bags deliver 100% oxygen directly to the patient, they can be used to deliver free-flow oxygen reliably at 100% concentration.

Flow-inflating bag

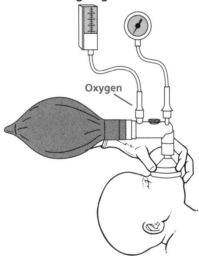

Figure 3.3. Flow-inflating bag

Advantages
- Delivers 100% oxygen at all times
- Easy to determine when there is a seal on the patient's face
- Stiffness of the lungs can be "felt" when squeezing the bag
- Can be used to deliver free-flow 100% oxygen

Disadvantages
- Requires a tight seal between the mask and the patient to remain inflated
- Requires a gas source to inflate
- Usually does not have a safety pop-off valve

The main disadvantage of using a flow-inflating bag is that it takes more practice to use effectively. Also, because it requires a gas source to inflate, it is sometimes not as quickly available for use when the need for resuscitation is unanticipated.

Since most flow-inflating bags do not have a safety valve, you may be more likely to overinflate the lungs unless you watch the degree of chest rise and the pressure manometer.

Self-inflating bag

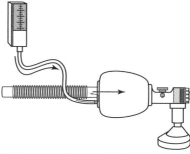

Figure 3.4. Self-inflating bag

Advantages
- Will always refill after being squeezed, even with no compressed gas source
- Pressure-release valve makes overinflation less likely

Disadvantages
- Will inflate even if there is not a seal between the mask and the patient's face
- Requires a reservoir attachment to deliver close to 100% oxygen
- Cannot be used to deliver 100% free-flow oxygen reliably

The self-inflating bag (Figure 3.4) is more commonly found in the hospital delivery room and resuscitation cart. It is somewhat easier to learn to use as it will refill after being squeezed, even if it is not attached to oxygen and even if its mask is not on a patient's face. The disadvantage of this, of course, is that you will be less likely to know if the oxygen line has become disconnected or if you have not achieved a good seal between the mask and the baby's face — both of which are necessary for effective resuscitation.

Even when the self-inflating bag is connected to a 100% oxygen source, some of the oxygen is directed out the back of the bag and an unpredictable amount is directed toward the patient unless the bag is being squeezed. When the bag is released, after being squeezed, the oxygen is diluted by room air, which is drawn in from the back of the bag unless an oxygen reservoir is in place. Therefore, a reservoir attachment is required to achieve 100% oxygen when the bag is being squeezed.

The amount of oxygen flow that comes out of the patient outlet of a self-inflating bag when the bag is not being squeezed is dependent on the relative resistance of several valves within the bag. Therefore, the bag will not reliably deliver 100% free-flow oxygen through the mask if it is not being squeezed.

You will learn that watching for chest movement is the most important sign of effective positive-pressure ventilation; if you watch for this important sign, bag-and-mask ventilation can be provided quite effectively with either type of bag.

What are the general characteristics of either type of resuscitation bag used to ventilate newborns?

The equipment should be specifically designed for newborns. Consideration should be given to the following:

• Size of bag

• Oxygen capability

• Safety features

• Size of mask

Size of bag no larger than 750 mL

Bags used for newborns should have a volume of 200 to 750 mL. Term newborns require only 15 to 25 mL with each ventilation (5 to 8 mL/kg). Bags larger than 750 mL, which are designed for older children and adults, make it difficult to provide such small volumes.

Capable of delivering 90% to 100% oxygen

Babies who require positive-pressure ventilation *at birth* should be ventilated initially with a high concentration of oxygen (90% to 100%). This can be accomplished by attaching a 100% oxygen source to either of the following:

• A flow-inflating bag

• A self-inflating bag with an oxygen reservoir

Note: Recent studies have suggested that babies can be successfully resuscitated with room air (21% oxygen). This supports the concept that ventilation is more important than high oxygen concentrations. However, the current recommendation is for 100% oxygen when it is available.

Capable of avoiding excessive pressures

To minimize complications resulting from high ventilation pressures, resuscitation bags should have certain safety features to prevent unwanted high pressures. These features will be different for each type of bag.

Appropriate-sized masks

A variety of mask sizes, appropriate for babies of different sizes, should be available at every delivery, since it is difficult to judge the appropriate size before birth. The mask should cover the chin, mouth, and nose, but not the eyes.

Each of these characteristics will be described later in this lesson.

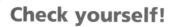

Check yourself!

(The answers are in the preceding section and at the end of the lesson.)

1. Flow-inflating bags (will) (will not) work without a compressed gas source.

2. A baby is born not breathing and blue. You have cleared his airway and stimulated him. Thirty seconds after birth, he has not improved. The next step is to (stimulate him more) (begin positive-pressure ventilation).

3. The single most important and most effective step in neonatal resuscitation is (stimulation) (ventilating the lungs).

4. Label these bags "flow-inflating" or "self-inflating."

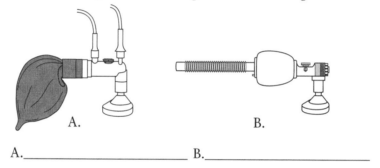

A. _____ B. _____

5. Neonatal ventilation bags are (much smaller than) (the same size as) adult ventilation bags.

6. Self-inflating bags require the attachment of a(n) _____ to deliver 100% oxygen.

7. Masks of different sizes (do) (do not) need to be available at every delivery.

What type of resuscitation bag is available in your hospital?

Find out what kind of resuscitation bag-and-mask device is used in your hospital. The characteristics and use of both the flow-inflating and the self-inflating bags will be described in this lesson. You will be responsible for knowing the general characteristics of both types of bags. However, you will need to know the details of, and should practice with, the one you use most frequently.

If you are required to learn the details of only the self-inflating bags, skip to page 3-13. Otherwise, continue with the text below.

Flow-inflating resuscitation bags

What are the parts of a flow-inflating bag?
There are four parts to a flow-inflating bag (Figure 3.5).
1. Oxygen inlet
2. Patient outlet
3. Flow-control valve
4. Pressure manometer attachment site

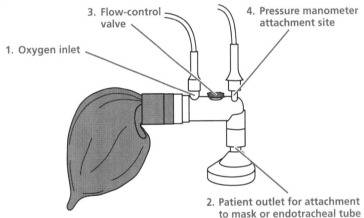

3. Flow-control valve

1. Oxygen inlet

4. Pressure manometer attachment site

2. Patient outlet for attachment to mask or endotracheal tube

Oxygen from a compressed source enters the bag at the *oxygen inlet*. The inlet is a small projection designed to fit oxygen tubing. The inlet may be at either end of the bag, depending on the brand and model you use.

Oxygen exits from the bag to the patient at the *patient outlet*, where the mask or endotracheal tube attaches to the bag.

The *flow-control valve* provides an adjustable leak that allows you to regulate the pressure in the bag when the bag is connected to an endotracheal tube or the mask is held tightly on the patient's face. The adjustable opening provides an additional outlet for the incoming oxygen and allows excess oxygen to escape rather than overinflate the bag or be forced into the patient.

Flow-inflating bags often have a *site for attaching a pressure manometer* (Figure 3.6). The attachment site is usually close to the patient outlet. The pressure manometer, as you will learn later, alerts you to the amount of pressure you are using to ventilate the newborn. If your flow-inflating bag has a connecting site for a pressure manometer, a manometer *must* be attached to the site. If the manometer is absent, the attachment site *must* be occluded with a plug or the site will be a source of leak and the bag will not inflate properly.

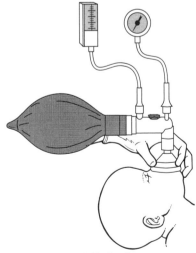

Figure 3.6. Flow-inflating bag attached to oxygen source and pressure manometer

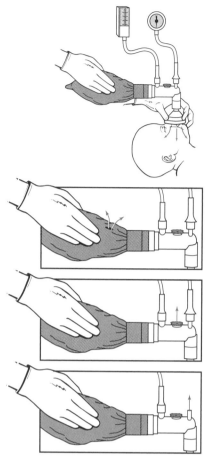

How does a flow-inflating bag work?
Since the inflation of the bag depends on a sealed system, the bag will not inflate if

• The mask is not properly sealed.

• There is a tear in the bag.

• The flow-control valve is open too wide.

• The pressure manometer is not attached or the oxygen tubing has become disconnected or occluded.

Figure 3.7. Reasons for failure of the flow-inflating bag to inflate

How do you adjust the oxygen flow and pressure in a flow-inflating bag?
When using a flow-inflating bag, you inflate the bag with compressed oxygen. Once the oxygen enters the bag, it is not diluted as it is in a self-inflating bag (as you will learn later). Therefore, whatever concentration of oxygen you put in the bag is the *same* concentration delivered to the patient. If the tubing from the bag is connected to a source of 100% oxygen, either from a wall outlet or a tank, 100% oxygen will be delivered to the baby.

Once you seal the mask on the baby's face (or connect the bag to an endotracheal tube, as you will learn in Lesson 5), all of the oxygen coming from the wall or tank will be directed to the bag (and thus to the patient) and out the flow-control valve. This will cause the bag to inflate (Figure 3.8). There are two ways that you can adjust the pressure in the bag and thus the amount of inflation of the bag.

- By adjusting the flowmeter, you regulate how much oxygen enters the bag.

- By adjusting the flow-control valve, you regulate how much oxygen escapes from the bag.

The flowmeter and flow-control valve should be set so that the bag is inflated to the point where it is comfortable to manage and does not completely deflate with each ventilation (Figure 3.9).

An overinflated bag is difficult to manage and may deliver excessive pressure to the baby. An underinflated bag makes it difficult to achieve the desired inflation pressure (Figure 3.10). With practice, you will be able to make the necessary adjustments to achieve a balance. If there is an adequate seal between the baby's face and the mask, you should be able to maintain the appropriate amount of inflation with the flowmeter set at 5 to 10 L/min.

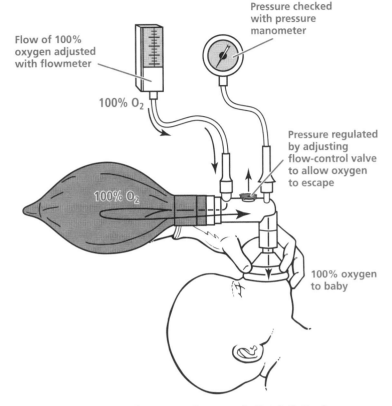

Flow of 100% oxygen adjusted with flowmeter

Pressure checked with pressure manometer

100% O₂

100% O₂

Pressure regulated by adjusting flow-control valve to allow oxygen to escape

100% oxygen to baby

Figure 3.8. Regulation of oxygen and pressure in flow-inflating bag

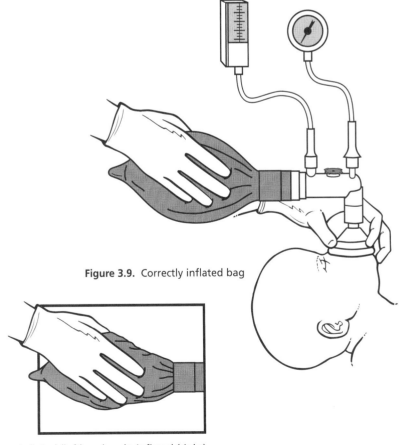

Figure 3.9. Correctly inflated bag

Figure 3.10. Resuscitation bags that are overinflated (left) and underinflated (right)

Check yourself!

(The answers are in the preceding section and at the end of the lesson.)

8. List four reasons why the flow-inflating bag may fail to ventilate the baby.

   (1)_____

   (2)_____

   (3)_____

   (4)_____

9. Which flow-inflating bag is being used properly?

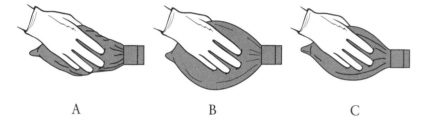

   A   B   C

10. To regulate the pressure of the oxygen going to the baby with a flow-inflating bag, you may adjust either the flowmeter on the wall or the (flow-control valve) (pressure manometer).

If you are required to learn the details of only the flow-inflating bag, skip to page 3-16. Otherwise, continue to the next page.

Self-inflating resuscitation bags

What are the parts of a self-inflating bag?
There are seven basic parts to a self-inflating bag (Figure 3.11).

1. Air inlet and attachment site for oxygen reservoir
2. Oxygen inlet
3. Patient outlet
4. Valve assembly
5. Oxygen reservoir
6. Pressure-release (pop-off) valve
7. Pressure manometer attachment site (optional)

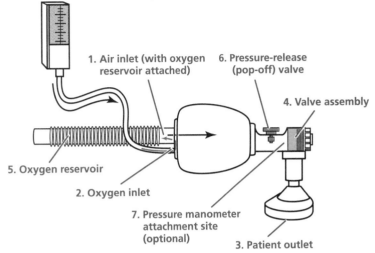

1. Air inlet (with oxygen reservoir attached)
6. Pressure-release (pop-off) valve
4. Valve assembly
5. Oxygen reservoir
2. Oxygen inlet
7. Pressure manometer attachment site (optional)
3. Patient outlet

Figure 3.11. Parts of a self-inflating bag

As the bag re-expands following compression, gas is drawn into the bag through a one-way valve that may be located at either end of the bag, depending on the design. This valve is called the *air inlet.*

Every self-inflating bag has an *oxygen inlet,* which usually is located near the air inlet. The oxygen inlet is a small nipple or projection to which oxygen tubing is attached. In the self-inflating bag, an oxygen tube does *not* need to be attached for the bag to function. The oxygen tube should be attached when the bag is to be used for neonatal resuscitation.

The *patient outlet* is where gas exits from the bag to the baby and where the mask or endotracheal tube attaches.

Self-inflating bags have a *valve assembly* positioned between the bag and the patient outlet (Figure 3.12). When the bag is squeezed during ventilation, the valve opens, releasing oxygen/air to the patient. When the bag reinflates (during the exhalation phase of the cycle), the valve is closed. This prevents the patient's exhaled air from entering the bag and being re-breathed. You should become familiar with the valve assembly — what it looks like and how it responds as you squeeze and release the bag. If it is missing or malfunctioning, the bag should not be used.

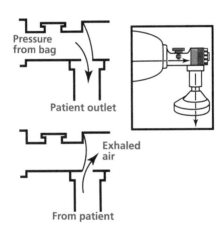

Pressure from bag

Patient outlet

Exhaled air

From patient

Figure 3.12. Principle of valve assembly of a self-inflating bag

Most self-inflating bags have a *pressure-release valve* that prevents excessive pressure build-up in the bag (Figure 3.11). Some self-inflating bags have a *site for attaching a pressure manometer.* The attachment site usually consists of a small hole or projection close to the patient outlet. If your bag has such a site, either the hole must be plugged or the manometer must be attached. Otherwise, gas will leak through the opening, preventing adequate pressure from being generated.

How do you control the oxygen and pressure in a self-inflating bag?
Current recommendations are that all babies who require resuscitation with assisted ventilation at birth should be ventilated with a high concentration of oxygen (90% to 100%). Oxygen can be brought into a self-inflating bag through tubing connected between an oxygen source and the oxygen inlet port on the bag. Each time the bag reinflates after you squeeze it, however, air is drawn into the bag through the air inlet. The air dilutes the concentration of oxygen in the bag. Therefore, even though you have 100% oxygen flowing through the oxygen inlet, it is diluted by the air that enters each time the bag reinflates. As a result, the concentration of oxygen actually received by the patient is greatly reduced to about 40% (Figure 3.13). Higher concentrations of oxygen should be used for resuscitating a baby at birth.

High concentrations of oxygen can be achieved with a self-inflating bag by using an *oxygen reservoir*. An oxygen reservoir is an appliance that can be placed over the bag's air inlet (Figure 3.14). The reservoir allows 100% oxygen to collect at the air inlet, thus preventing the oxygen from being diluted with room air. However, the flow of oxygen is delivered reliably to the patient only when the bag is squeezed.

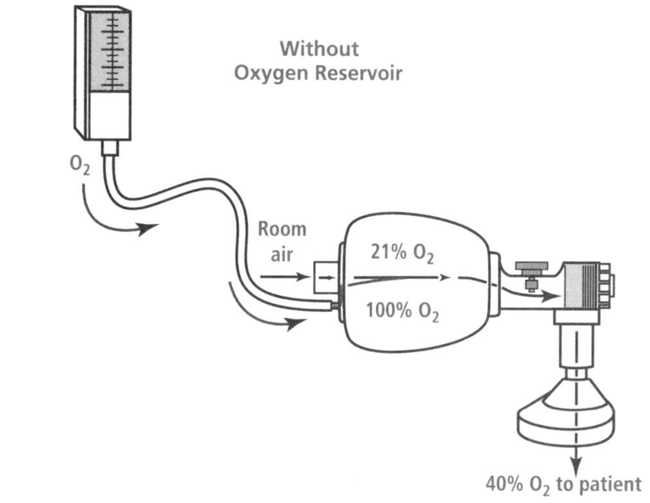

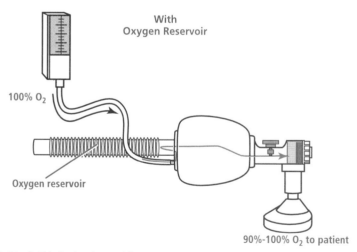

Figure 3.13. Self-inflating bag without an oxygen reservoir delivers only 40% oxygen to the patient

Figure 3.14. Self-inflating bag with oxygen reservoir delivers 90% to 100% oxygen to the patient

There are several different types of oxygen reservoirs, but they all perform the same function. Some have open ends and others have a valve that allows some air to enter the reservoir (Figure 3.15). Therefore, the concentration of oxygen achieved with a self-inflating bag with an oxygen reservoir attached will be between 90% and 100%.

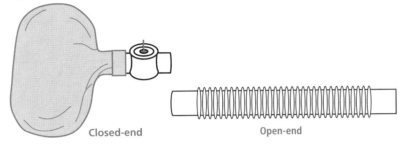

Closed-end   Open-end

Figure 3.15. Different types of oxygen reservoirs for self-inflating bags

The amount of pressure delivered by a self-inflating bag is *not* dependent on the flow of oxygen entering the bag. When you seal the mask on the baby's face (or connect the bag to an endotracheal tube), there will be no change in the inflation of a self-inflating bag. The amount of pressure and volume delivered with each breath depends on the following three factors:

• How hard you squeeze the bag

• Any leak that may be present between the mask and the baby's face

• The set-point of the pressure-release valve (as described later in this lesson)

Check yourself!

(The answers are in the preceding section and at the end of the lesson.)

11. A self-inflating bag with a pressure manometer site will work only if a pressure manometer is connected to the site or if the connection site is (left open) (plugged).

12. A self-inflating bag can deliver 90% to 100% oxygen (by itself) (only when an oxygen reservoir is attached to it).

13. A self-inflating bag connected to 100% oxygen, but without an oxygen reservoir attached to it, can deliver only about _____% oxygen.

14. The pressure delivered from a self-inflating bag is determined by what three factors?
    (1)_____
    (2)_____
    (3)_____

What safety features are there to prevent the pressure in the bag from getting too high?

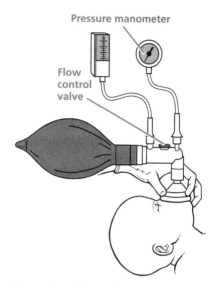

Pressure manometer

Flow control valve

You will attach a resuscitation bag to either a mask, which will be held tight on the patient's face, or to an endotracheal tube, which will be in the patient's trachea. In either case, if you ventilate with excessive pressure, the lungs could become overinflated, thus causing rupture of the alveoli and a resulting air leak, such as a pneumothorax.

Figure 3.16. Flow-inflating bag with flow-control valve and pressure manometer

 Any resuscitation bag, whether it is flow-inflating or self-inflating, should be equipped with one or both of the following safety features to prevent the development of excessive pressure:

- **Pressure manometer and flow-control valve (Figure 3.16)**
- **Pressure-release valve (Figure 3.17)**

Flow-inflating bags have the flow-control valve, which can be adjusted to deliver the desired peak pressure. A pressure manometer attached to the bag will allow you to properly adjust the valve.

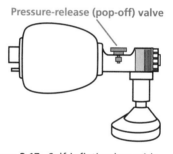

Pressure-release (pop-off) valve

Self-inflating bags should have a pressure-release valve (commonly called a *pop-off valve*), which is generally set to 30 to 40 cm H_2O. If pressures greater than 30 to 40 cm H_2O are generated, the valve opens, limiting the pressure being transmitted to the newborn. There may be wide variation in the point at which a pressure-release valve opens. The make and age of the bag as well as the method with which it has been cleaned affect the opening pressure of the valve.

Figure 3.17. Self-inflating bag with pressure-release (pop-off) valve

In some self-inflating bags, the pressure-release valve can be temporarily occluded or bypassed to allow high pressures to be administered. This may occasionally be necessary to ventilate a newborn's non-aerated lungs, especially with the first few breaths. Extreme care must be taken not to use excessive pressure during the first few ventilations while the pressure-release valve is bypassed. Many self-inflating bags are also equipped with a port to attach a pressure manometer.

 Be certain to connect the oxygen supply line to the correct connection site as indicated by the bag's manufacturer. Connection to the wrong port has been reported to result in inadvertent high pressures being delivered to the patient.

Can you give free-flow oxygen using a bag and mask?

Yes, with a flow-inflating bag.

A flow-inflating bag and mask can be used to deliver free-flow oxygen (Figure 3.18). The mask should be loosely placed on the face, allowing some gas to escape around the edges. If the mask is held tightly to the face, pressure will build up in the bag and be transmitted to the newborn's lungs. The bag should not inflate when used to provide free-flow oxygen. An inflated bag indicates that the mask is tight against the face and positive pressure is being provided.

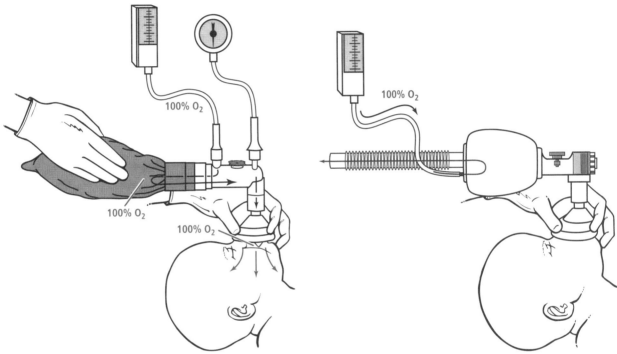

Figure 3.18. Free-flow 100% oxygen given by flow-inflating bag. Note that mask is not held tight on face.

Figure 3.19. Free-flow 100% oxygen *cannot* be given reliably by self-inflating bag; bag must be squeezed for reliable 90% to 100% oxygen delivery.

No, with a self-inflating bag.

Free-flow oxygen *cannot* be given reliably with a self-inflating bag-and-mask device.

The oxygen flow entering a self-inflating bag will normally be diverted to the air inlet, through its attached oxygen reservoir, and then evacuated either out the end of the oxygen reservoir or out a valve that is attached to the reservoir (Figure 3.19). The amount of oxygen sent to the patient will depend on the relative resistance of the various valves and, therefore, may not reach the patient unless the bag is being squeezed. If your hospital is equipped with self-inflating bags, you may need to have a separate set-up available for delivering free-flow oxygen, as described in Lesson 2.

Figure 3.20. Face masks with cushioned rims

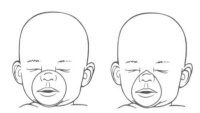

Figure 3.21. Round (left) and anatomically shaped (right) face masks

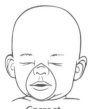

Correct
Covers mouth, nose, and chin but not eyes

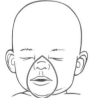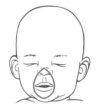

Incorrect
Too large: covers eyes and extends over chin

Incorrect
Too small: does not cover nose and mouth well

Figure 3.22. Correct (top) and incorrect (bottom) mask sizes

What characteristics of face masks make them most effective for ventilating newborns?

Masks come in a variety of shapes, sizes, and materials. Selection of a mask for use with a particular newborn will depend on how well the mask fits the newborn's face and how easy it is to conform to the face and obtain a seal with it.

Resuscitation masks have rims that are either *cushioned* or *noncushioned.*

The rim on a *cushioned* mask (Figure 3.20) is made from either a soft, flexible material, such as foam rubber, or an air-inflated ring. A cushioned-rim mask has several advantages over a mask without a cushioned rim.

- The rim conforms more easily to the shape of the newborn's face, making it easier to form a seal.
- It requires less pressure on the newborn's face to obtain a seal.
- There is less chance of damaging the newborn's eyes if the mask is incorrectly positioned.

Some masks are constructed without a padded, soft rim. Such a mask usually has a very firm edge to the rim. A mask with a noncushioned rim can cause several problems.

- It is more difficult to obtain a seal, because it does not easily conform to the shape of the baby's face.
- It can damage the eyes if the mask is improperly positioned.
- It can bruise the newborn's face if the mask is applied too firmly.

Masks also come in two shapes: round and anatomically shaped (Figure 3.21). Anatomically shaped masks are shaped to fit the contours of the face. They are made to be placed on the face with the most pointed part of the mask fitting over the nose.

Masks also come in several sizes. Masks suitable for small premature babies as well as for term babies should be available for use.

For the mask to be the correct size, the rim will cover the tip of the chin, the mouth, and the nose but not the eyes (Figure 3.22).

- Too large — may cause possible eye damage and will not seal well
- Too small — will not cover the mouth and nose and may occlude the nose

PREMATURITY POINTERS

Be sure to have very small masks available if a preterm delivery is expected. Extremely low-birthweight babies are often difficult to ventilate by bag and mask, which is one reason that they are often intubated early in the course of a resuscitation.

What should be done to prepare the equipment for an anticipated resuscitation?

Assemble equipment
The bag should be assembled and connected to oxygen so that it will provide the necessary 90% to 100% concentration. If a self-inflating bag is used, be sure the oxygen reservoir is attached. Anticipate the size of the baby at delivery, and be sure you have appropriate-sized masks. Check the masks carefully for any cracks or defects in the rim.

Test the equipment
Once the equipment has been selected and assembled, check the bag and mask to be sure they function properly. Success in using a bag and mask requires more than up-to-date equipment and a skilled operator — the equipment must be in working order. Bags that have cracks or tears, valves that stick or leak, or masks that are cracked or deflated must not be used. The equipment should be checked before each delivery. The operator should check it again just before its use. Since there are different things to check on a flow-inflating bag and a self-inflating bag, each type of bag will be discussed separately.

Testing a flow-inflating bag
To check a flow-inflating bag, attach it to a gas source. Adjust the flowmeter to 5 to 10 L/min. Block the patient outlet to make sure the bag fills properly (Figure 3.23). Do this by making a seal between the mask and the palm of your hand. (Some people prefer to remove the mask to more easily achieve a seal directly on the bag outlet.) Adjust the flow-control valve so that the bag is not over-distended. Watch the pressure manometer, and adjust the valve so that there is approximately 5 cm H_2O pressure when the bag is not being squeezed and 30 to 40 cm H_2O peak inflation pressure when the bag is squeezed firmly.

Does the bag fill properly? If not,

- Is there a crack or tear in the bag?
- Is the flow-control valve open too far?
- Is the pressure manometer attached?
- Is the oxygen line connected securely?
- Is the patient outlet sufficiently blocked?

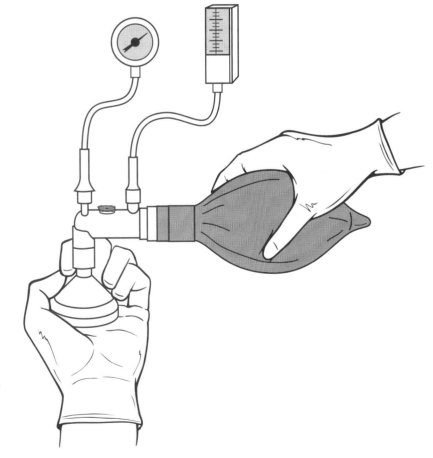

Figure 3.23. Testing a flow-inflating bag

If the bag fills, squeeze the bag.

- Do you feel pressure against your hand?
- Does the pressure manometer register under 5 cm H_2O pressure when not squeezed and 30 to 40 cm H_2O when squeezed firmly?

Squeeze the bag at a rate of 40 to 60 times per minute and pressures of 40 cm H_2O. If the bag does not fill rapidly enough, readjust the flow-control valve or increase the oxygen flow from the flowmeter.

If the bag still does not fill properly or does not generate adequate pressure, get another bag and begin again.

Testing a self-inflating bag
First, check to be certain that the oxygen tubing and oxygen reservoir are connected, and adjust the flow to 5 to 10 L/min (Figure 3.24).

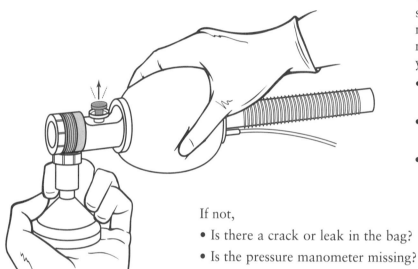

To check the operation of a self-inflating bag, block the mask or patient outlet by making a seal with the palm of your hand. Then squeeze the bag.

- Do you feel pressure against your hand?
- Can you force the pressure-release valve open?
- Does the pressure manometer (if present) register 30 to 40 cm H_2O pressure?

If not,

- Is there a crack or leak in the bag?
- Is the pressure manometer missing?
- Is the pressure-release valve missing or stuck closed?
- Is the patient outlet sufficiently blocked?

If your bag generates adequate pressure and the safety features are working while the mask-patient outlet is blocked,

- Does the bag reinflate quickly when you release your grip?

Figure 3.24. Testing a self-inflating bag

If there is any problem with the bag, obtain a new one. Self-inflating bags usually have more parts than flow-inflating bags. During cleaning, parts may be left out, assembled incorrectly, or left moist, causing them to stick.

 You should become very familiar with the type of bag you are using. You must know exactly how to check it to quickly determine whether it is functioning properly.

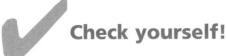

✔ Check yourself!

(The answers are in the preceding section and at the end of the lesson.)

15. Free-flow oxygen can be delivered reliably only with a (flow-inflating bag) (self-inflating bag).

16. When giving free-flow oxygen with a bag and mask, it is necessary to place the mask (securely) (loosely) on the baby's face to allow some gas to escape around the edges of the mask.

17. Which mask is the correct size?

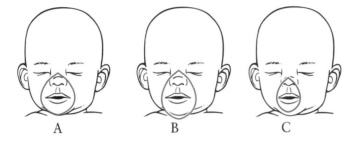

     A   B   C

18. Before an anticipated resuscitation, the ventilation bag should be connected to a(n) _____.

19. When you test a resuscitation bag, you (make) (do not make) an airtight seal between the mask and the palm of your hand.

20. When you test a flow-inflating bag, you watch to see if the bag (inflates) (deflates).

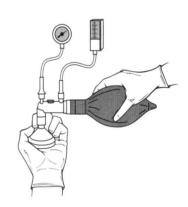

21. You are testing a resuscitation bag. When you squeeze the bag you (should) (should not) feel pressure against your hand.

22. If the resuscitation bag on the right is working properly, what should the pressure manometer read when you squeeze the bag?

_____

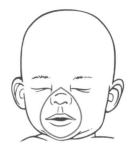

Figure 3.25. Correct-sized mask covers mouth, nose, and tip of chin, but not the eyes

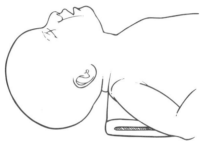

Figure 3.26. Correct position for assisted ventilation

What do you need to check before assisting ventilation with a resuscitation bag?

Select the appropriate-sized mask.
Remember, the mask should cover the mouth, nose, and tip of the chin, but not the eyes (Figure 3.25).

Be sure there is a clear airway.
You may want to suction the mouth and nose one more time to be certain there will be no obstruction to the assisted breaths that you will be delivering.

Position the baby's head.
As described in Lesson 2, the baby's neck should be slightly extended (but not overextended) to maintain an open airway. One way to accomplish this is to place a small roll under the shoulders (Figure 3.26).

If the baby's position has shifted, reposition the baby before continuing.

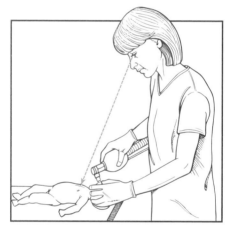 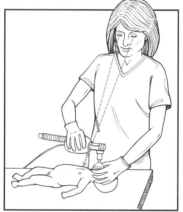

Figure 3.27. Two correct positions for visualizing chest movement during assisted ventilation

Position yourself at the bedside.
You also will need to position yourself at the side or head of the baby to use the resuscitation bag effectively (Figure 3.27). This position will allow you to hold the mask on the baby's face comfortably. If you are right-handed, you probably will feel most comfortable controlling the bag with your right hand and the mask with your left hand. If you are left-handed, you will probably want to control the bag with your left hand and hold the mask with your right hand. The mask may be swiveled on the bag for optimum fit to the face and to your position.

It is important that the bag is positioned so that it does not block your view of the baby's chest, since you need to be able to observe the rise and fall of the chest during ventilation.

Both positions leave the chest and abdomen unobstructed for visual monitoring of the baby, for chest compressions, and for vascular access via the umbilical cord should these procedures become necessary.

How do you position the bag and mask on the face?

The mask should be placed on the face so that it covers the nose and mouth, and the tip of the chin rests within the rim of the mask. You may find it helpful to begin by cupping the chin in the mask and then covering the nose (Figure 3.28).

The mask usually is held on the face with the thumb, index, and/or middle finger encircling much of the rim of the mask, while the ring and fifth fingers bring the chin forward to maintain a patient airway.

Remember, anatomically shaped masks should be positioned with the pointed end over the nose. Once the mask is positioned, an airtight seal can be formed by using *light* downward pressure on the rim of the mask.

Care should be taken in holding the mask. Observe the following precautions:

- Do not "jam" the mask down on the face. Too much pressure can mold (flatten) the back of the head and bruise the face.

- Do not allow your fingers or parts of your hand to rest on the baby's eyes.

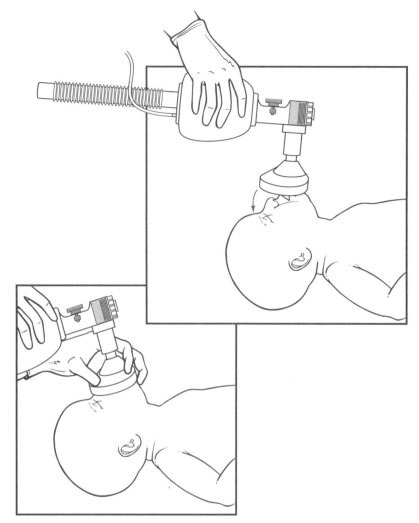

Figure 3.28. Correctly positioning mask on the face

Why is establishing a seal between the mask and the face so important?

An airtight seal between the rim of the mask and the face is essential to achieve the positive pressure required to inflate the lungs.

Also, a flow-inflating bag will not stay inflated without a good mask-face seal and, therefore, you won't be able to squeeze the bag to create the desired pressure.

Although a self-inflating bag will remain inflated despite an inadequate seal, when you squeeze the bag you will not be able to generate pressure to inflate the lungs.

Remember

- A tight seal is required for a flow-inflating bag to inflate.
- A tight seal is required for either type of bag to generate positive pressure to inflate the lungs when it is squeezed.

How do you know how hard to squeeze the bag?

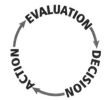

A noticeable rise and fall of the chest is by far the best indication that the mask is sealed and the lungs are being inflated. The newborn should appear to be taking a normal or "easy" breath.

The presence of bilateral breath sounds and improvement of the baby's color and heart rate are other indications that the newborn is being properly ventilated.

Remember, the lungs of a fetus are filled with fluid, but the lungs of a newborn must be filled with air. In order to establish a gaseous volume (functional residual capacity) in the newly born baby, the first few breaths will often require higher pressures and longer inflation times than will subsequent breaths. This requirement for increased and more prolonged pressure is more likely to be found in a baby who is not breathing spontaneously.

If you have a pressure manometer connected to the bag, you can look at the actual pressure you are delivering. Although you should ventilate with the lowest pressure required to move the chest adequately, initial breaths may require pressures of more than 30 cm H_2O. Subsequent breaths usually require less pressure.

Illustrative pressures
- Initial breath after delivery   >30 cm H_2O
- Normal lungs (later breaths)   15 to 20 cm H_2O
- Diseased or immature lungs   20 to 40 cm H_2O

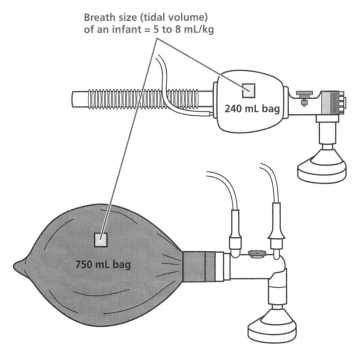

Breath size (tidal volume) of an infant = 5 to 8 mL/kg

240 mL bag

750 mL bag

Figure 3.29. Relative sizes of a normal breath and common resuscitation bags

If the baby appears to be taking a very deep breath, the lungs are being overinflated. You are using too much pressure, and there is danger of producing a pneumothorax. Remember that the volume of a normal newborn breath is much smaller than the amount of gas in your resuscitation bag: one tenth of a 240-mL self-inflating bag; one thirtieth of a 750-mL flow-inflating bag (Figure 3.29).

Abdominal movement may be misleading. Abdominal movement may be due to air entering the stomach and can be mistaken for effective ventilation.

PREMATURITY POINTERS
Premature babies have even smaller breath sizes, with some as small as 5 to 10 mL. However, they may also have stiffer lungs, thus requiring higher inflation pressures to deliver these smaller volumes.

How often should you squeeze the bag?

During the initial stages of neonatal resuscitation, breaths should be delivered at a rate of *40 to 60 breaths per minute,* or slightly less than once a second.

To help maintain a rate of 40 to 60 breaths per minute, try saying to yourself as you ventilate the newborn

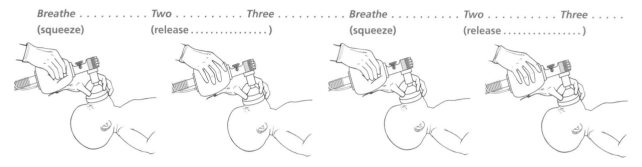

Breathe . . . . Two . . . . Three . . . . Breathe . . . . Two . . . . Three . . . . .
(squeeze)   (release . . . .)   (squeeze)   (release . . . .)

Figure 3.30. Counting out loud to maintain a rate of 40 to 60 breaths per minute

If you squeeze the bag on "Breathe" and release while you say "Two, Three," you will probably find you are ventilating at a proper rate (Figure 3.30).

What do you do if the chest is not rising with each squeeze of the bag?

If the chest does not expand adequately, it may be due to one or more of the following reasons:

• The seal is inadequate.

• The airway is blocked.

• Not enough pressure is being given.

Inadequate seal
If you hear or feel air escaping from around the mask, reapply the mask to the face and try to form a better seal. Use a little more pressure on the rim of the mask. *Do not* press down hard on the baby's face. The most common place for a leak to occur is between the cheek and bridge of the nose (Figure 3.31).

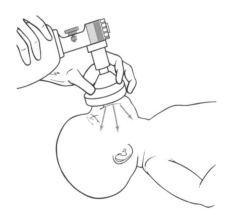

Figure 3.31. Inadequate seal of mask on face may result in poor chest rise

Blocked airway
Another possible reason for insufficient ventilation of the baby's lungs is a blocked airway. To correct this,

• Check the baby's position and extend the neck a bit farther.

• Check the mouth, oropharynx, and nose for secretions; suction the mouth and nose if necessary.

• Try ventilating with the baby's mouth slightly open (especially helpful in extremely small premature babies with very small nares).

Not enough pressure

You may be squeezing the bag with inadequate pressure.

- Increase the pressure. If using a bag with a *pressure manometer,* note the amount of pressure required to result in adequate chest rise.

- If using a bag with a *pressure-release valve,* increase the pressure until the valve actuates. If more pressure is required and it is possible to occlude the pressure-release valve, do so, and cautiously increase the pressure.

- If adequate chest rise still cannot be achieved, endotracheal intubation may be required.

In summary, if you do not observe chest expansion, try the following steps until the chest expands:

Condition	Actions
1. Inadequate seal	Reapply mask to face.
2. Blocked airway	Reposition the head.
	Check for secretions; suction if present.
	Ventilate with newborn's mouth slightly open.
3. Not enough pressure	Increase pressure until there is an easy rise and fall of the chest
	Consider endotracheal intubation.

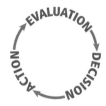

If you still are unable to obtain adequate chest expansion after going through this sequence, endotracheal intubation and bag-and-tube ventilation will usually be required.

How do you know if the baby is improving and that you can stop positive-pressure ventilation?

Improvement is indicated by three signs.

- Increasing heart rate
- Improving color
- Spontaneous breathing

The steps you go through will depend on the degree of improvement in the newborn's condition.

As the heart rate keeps increasing toward normal, you should continue ventilating the baby at a rate of 40 to 60 breaths per minute. Monitor the rise of the chest to prevent overinflation or underinflation of the lungs. With improvement, the baby also should become pink.

When the heart rate stabilizes above 100 bpm, the rates and pressure of assisted ventilation should be reduced gradually while you stimulate the baby to breathe. Continue to provide 100% oxygen while stimulating and observing for spontaneous respirations.

If the baby is breathing spontaneously and the heart rate has reached an acceptable level, you may discontinue assisted ventilation as the rate and depth of spontaneous respirations become adequate. Free-flow oxygen should be continued as necessary to keep the baby pink.

✔ Check yourself!

(The answers are in the preceding section and at the end of the lesson.)

23. Which baby is positioned properly for ventilation with a resuscitation bag?

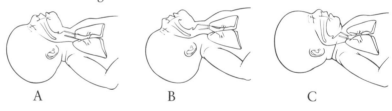

A   B   C

24. Which illustration(s) shows the correct position for assisting ventilation with a resuscitation bag?

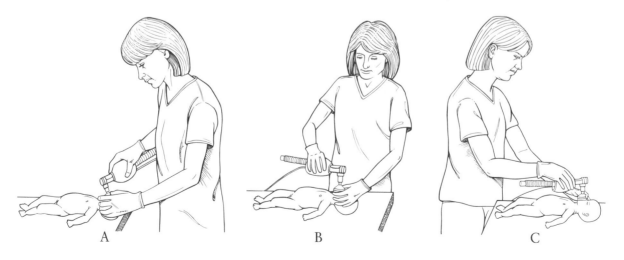

A   B   C

25. You must hold the resuscitation bag so that you can see the newborn's _____ and _____.

26. An anatomically shaped mask should be positioned with the (pointed) (rounded) end over the newborn's nose.

27. You are using a self-inflating bag to ventilate a baby. The bag fills after every squeeze. You look to see if the baby's chest is rising with each breath, and it is not. List three possibilities of what may be wrong.
    (1)_____
    (2)_____
    (3)_____

28. If you notice that the baby's chest looks as if he is taking deep breaths, you are (overinflating) (underinflating) the lungs, and there is danger you will produce a pneumothorax.

29. When ventilating a baby, you should squeeze the resuscitation bag at a rate of _____ to _____ breaths per minute.

30. If, after making appropriate adjustments, you are unable to obtain chest expansion with bag-and-mask ventilation, you will usually have to insert a(n) _____ and begin bag-and- _____ ventilation.

31. You notice that a baby's chest is moving as you ventilate him. Another way to check for good aeration is to use a(n) _____ to listen for _____ sounds in both lungs.

32. Before stopping assisted ventilation, you should (increase) (decrease) the rate and check the following three physical signs:
    (1)_____
    (2)_____
    (3)_____

Is there anything else to do if bag-and-mask ventilation is to be continued for more than several minutes?

Newborns requiring bag-and-mask ventilation for longer than several minutes should have an orogastric tube inserted and left in place.

During bag-and-mask ventilation, gas is forced into the oropharynx, where it is free to enter both the trachea and the esophagus. Proper positioning of the newborn will transmit most of the air into the trachea and the lungs. However, some gas may enter the esophagus and be forced into the stomach (Figure 3.32).

Gas forced into the stomach interferes with ventilation in the following ways:

• A stomach distended with gas puts pressure on the diaphragm, preventing full expansion of the lungs.

• Gas in the stomach may cause regurgitation of gastric contents, which may then be aspirated during bag-and-mask ventilation.

The problems related to gastric/abdominal distention and aspiration of gastric contents can be reduced by inserting an orogastric tube, suctioning gastric contents, and leaving the gastric tube in place to act as a vent for gas throughout the remainder of the resuscitation.

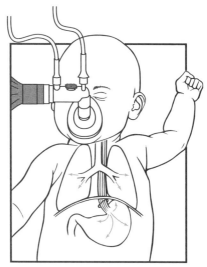

Figure 3.32. Excess gas in stomach resulting from bag-and-mask ventilation

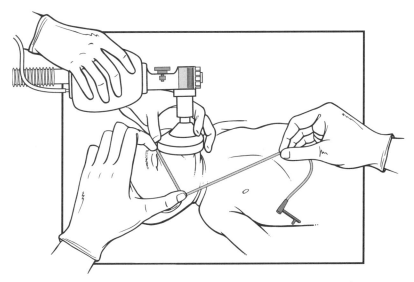

Figure 3.33. Measuring the correct distance for inserting an orogastric tube

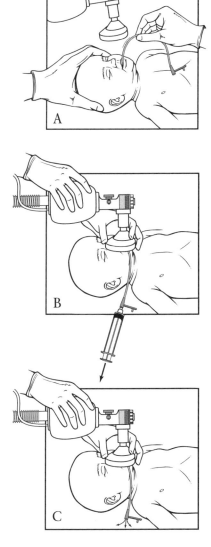

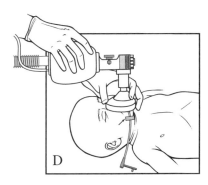

Figure 3.34. Insertion, aspiration, and taping of an orogastric tube (top to bottom)

How do you insert an orogastric tube?

The equipment you will need to place an orogastric tube during ventilation includes

- 8F feeding tube
- 20-mL syringe

The major steps are as follows:

1. Always measure the length of the tube you want to insert. It must be long enough to reach the stomach but not so long as to bypass beyond it. The length of the inserted tube should be equal to *the distance from the bridge of the nose to the earlobe and from the earlobe to the xyphoid process* (the lower tip of the sternum). Note the centimeter mark at this place on the tube (Figure 3.33).

    To minimize interruption of ventilation, measurement of the orogastric tube can be approximated with the mask in place.

2. Insert the tube through the **mouth** rather than the nose (Figure 3.34A). The nose should be left open for ventilation. Ventilation can be resumed as soon as the tube has been placed.

3. Once the tube is inserted the desired distance, attach a syringe and quickly but gently remove the gastric contents (Figure 3.34B).

4. Remove the syringe from the tube and leave the end of the tube *open* to provide a vent for air entering the stomach (Figure 3.34C).

5. Tape the tube to the baby's cheek to ensure that the tip remains in the stomach and is not pulled back into the esophagus (Figure 3.34D).

    The tube will not interfere with the mask-to-face seal if an 8F feeding tube is used and the tube exits from the side of the mask over the soft area of the baby's cheek. A larger tube may make it difficult to obtain a seal. A smaller tube can easily become occluded by secretions.

What do you do if the baby is *not* improving?

The vast majority of babies requiring resuscitation will improve if given adequate positive-pressure ventilation. Therefore, you should ensure that the lungs are being adequately ventilated with 100% oxygen.

Is chest movement adequate?

Check for adequacy of chest expansion, and use a stethoscope to listen for bilateral breath sounds.

- Is the face-mask seal tight?
- Is the airway blocked because of improper head position or secretions in the nose, mouth, or pharynx?
- Is the bag working properly?
- Is adequate pressure being used?
- Is air in the stomach interfering with chest expansion?

Is 100% oxygen being administered?

- Is the oxygen tubing attached to the bag *and* to the oxygen source?
- Is gas flowing through the flowmeter?
- If using a self-inflating bag, is the oxygen reservoir attached?
- If using a tank (rather than wall oxygen), is there oxygen in the tank?

These all seem obvious. However, in the urgency created by a newborn needing resuscitation, some of these points may be overlooked.

Bag-and-mask ventilation generally is not as effective as bag-and-endotracheal-tube ventilation because with bag and mask, some of the positive pressure will escape down the esophagus into the stomach.

Therefore, if you have checked all of these factors and chest expansion is still not satisfactory, or if you don't hear good breath sounds bilaterally, it usually will be appropriate to insert an endotracheal tube at this time. This procedure will be described in Lesson 5.

Complications, such as a pneumothorax, also may have occurred. These will be described in Lesson 7.

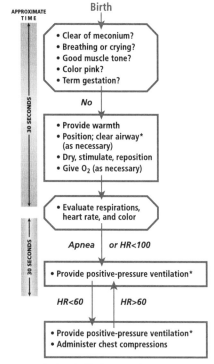

APPROXIMATE TIME

Birth

30 SECONDS

- Clear of meconium?
- Breathing or crying?
- Good muscle tone?
- Color pink?
- Term gestation?

No

- Provide warmth
- Position; clear airway* (as necessary)
- Dry, stimulate, reposition
- Give O₂ (as necessary)

30 SECONDS

- Evaluate respirations, heart rate, and color

Apnea | or HR<100

- Provide positive-pressure ventilation*

HR<60 | HR>60

- Provide positive-pressure ventilation*
- Administer chest compressions

*Endotracheal intubation may be considered at several steps.

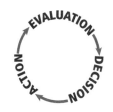

Remember, establishing effective ventilation is the key to nearly all successful neonatal resuscitations.

If the baby's condition continues to deteriorate or fails to improve, and the heart rate is less than 60 bpm despite 30 seconds of adequate positive-pressure ventilation, your next step will be to begin chest compressions. This will be described in the next lesson.

Lesson 3 Review

(The answers are at the end of the lesson.)

1. Flow-inflating bags (will) (will not) work without a compressed gas source.

2. A baby is born not breathing and blue. You have cleared his airway and stimulated him. Thirty seconds after birth, he has not improved. The next step is to (stimulate him more) (begin positive-pressure ventilation).

3. The single most important and most effective step in neonatal resuscitation is (stimulation) (ventilating the lungs).

4. Label these bags "flow-inflating" or "self-inflating."

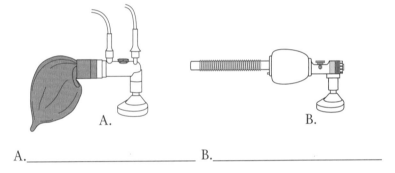

   A.   B.

   A._____ B._____

5. Neonatal ventilation bags are (much smaller than) (the same size as) adult ventilation bags.

6. Self-inflating bags require the attachment of a(n) _____ to deliver 100% oxygen.

7. Masks of different sizes (do) (do not) need to be available at every delivery.

If you are required to learn only the self-inflating bag, skip to question 11.

Lesson 3 Review — *continued*

(The answers are at the end of the lesson.)

8. List four reasons why the flow-inflating bag may fail to ventilate the baby.

   (1)_____

   (2)_____

   (3)_____

   (4)_____

9. Which flow-inflating bag is being used properly?

   A   B   C

10. To regulate the pressure of the oxygen going to the baby with a flow-inflating bag, you may adjust either the flowmeter on the wall or the (flow-control valve) (pressure manometer).

If you are required to learn only the flow-inflating bag, skip to question 15.

11. A self-inflating bag with a pressure manometer site will work only if a pressure manometer is connected to the site or if the connection site is (left open) (plugged).

12. A self-inflating bag can deliver 90% to 100% oxygen (by itself) (only when an oxygen reservoir is attached to it).

13. A self-inflating bag connected to 100% oxygen, but without an oxygen reservoir attached to it, can deliver only about ____% oxygen.

14. The pressure delivered from a self-inflating bag is determined by what three factors?

    (1)_____

    (2)_____

    (3)_____

Lesson 3 Review — *continued*

(The answers are at the end of the lesson.)

15. Free-flow oxygen can be delivered reliably only with a (flow-inflating bag) (self-inflating bag).

16. When giving free-flow oxygen with a bag and mask, it is necessary to place the mask (securely) (loosely) on the baby's face to allow some gas to escape around the edges of the mask.

17. Which mask is the correct size?

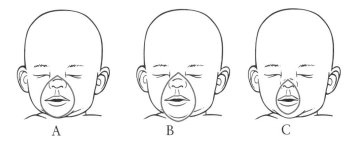

A   B   C

18. Before an anticipated resuscitation, the ventilation bag should be connected to a(n) _____.

19. When you test a resuscitation bag, you (make) (do not make) an airtight seal between the mask and the palm of your hand.

20. When you test a flow-inflating bag, you watch to see if the bag (inflates) (deflates).

21. You are testing a resuscitation bag. When you squeeze the bag you (should) (should not) feel pressure against your hand.

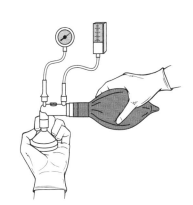

22. If the resuscitation bag on the right is working properly, what should the pressure manometer read when you squeeze the bag?

_____

23. Which baby is positioned properly for ventilation with a resuscitation bag?

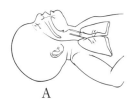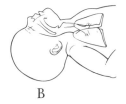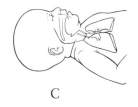

A   B   C

Lesson 3 Review — *continued*

(The answers are at the end of the lesson.)

24. Which illustration(s) shows the correct position for assisting ventilation with a resuscitation bag?

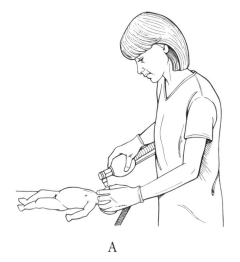 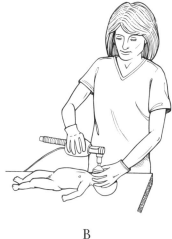 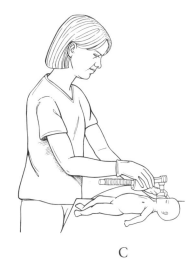

       A   B   C

25. You must hold the resuscitation bag so that you can see the newborn's _____ and _____.

26. An anatomically shaped mask should be positioned with the (pointed) (rounded) end over the newborn's nose.

27. You are using a self-inflating bag to ventilate a baby. The bag fills after every squeeze. You look to see if the baby's chest is rising with each breath, and it is not. List three possibilities of what may be wrong.
    (1)_____
    (2)_____
    (3)_____

28. If you notice that the baby's chest looks as if he is taking deep breaths, you are (overinflating) (underinflating) the lungs, and there is danger you will produce a pneumothorax.

29. When ventilating a baby, you should squeeze the resuscitation bag at a rate of _____ to _____ breaths per minute.

3

Lesson 3 Review — *continued*

(The answers are at the end of the lesson.)

30. If, after making appropriate adjustments, you are unable to obtain chest expansion with bag-and-mask ventilation, you will usually have to insert a(n) _____ and begin bag-and- _____ ventilation.

31. You notice that a baby's chest is moving as you ventilate him. Another way to check for good aeration is to use a(n) _____ to listen for _____ sounds in both lungs.

32. Before stopping assisted ventilation, you should (increase) (decrease) the rate and check the following three physical signs:
    (1)_____
    (2)_____
    (3)_____

33. If you must continue bag-and-mask ventilation for more than several minutes, a(n) _____ should be inserted to act as a vent for the gas in the stomach during the remainder of the resuscitation.

34. How far should this orogastric catheter be inserted? _____cm

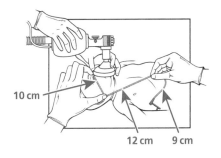

10 cm   12 cm   9 cm

35. As soon as the orogastric catheter is inserted, a syringe is attached and gastric contents are removed. Then the syringe is removed, and the catheter is left _____ to vent stomach gas.

36. After the orogastric catheter has been inserted, bag-and-mask ventilation (should) (should not) continue.

37. The vast majority of babies requiring resuscitation (will) (will not) improve with positive-pressure ventilation by bag and mask.

Performance Checklist
Lesson 3 — Bag-and-Mask Ventilation

Instructor: The learner should be instructed to talk through the procedure as it is demonstrated. Judge the performance of each step and check (✓) the box when the action is completed correctly. If done incorrectly, circle the box so that you can discuss that step later. You will need to provide information at several points concerning the condition of the baby.

Learner: To successfully complete this checklist, you should be able to perform all the steps and make all the correct decisions in the procedure. You should talk through the procedure as you perform it.

Equipment and Supplies

Newborn resuscitation manikin

Radiant warmer or table to simulate warmer

Gloves (or may simulate this)

Bulb syringe or suction catheter

Stethoscope

Shoulder roll

Self-inflating bag

    or

Flow-inflating bag with pressure manometer and oxygen source

Flowmeter (or may simulate this)

Masks (term and preterm sizes)

Method to administer free-flow oxygen (oxygen mask, oxygen tubing, or flow-inflating bag and mask)

Feeding tube and syringe

Tape

Clock with second hand

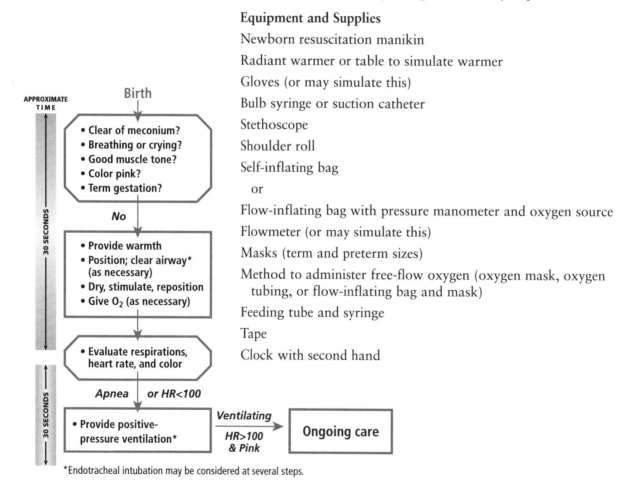

*Endotracheal intubation may be considered at several steps.

Performance Checklist
Lesson 3 — Bag-and-Mask Ventilation

Name _____ Instructor _____ Date _____

Instructor's questions are in quotes. Learner's questions and correct responses are in bold type. Instructor should check boxes as the learner answers correctly.

"You are called to the delivery of a baby with an estimated gestation of ____ weeks. How would you prepare the ventilation equipment for this baby? You may ask me anything you would like to know about the baby's condition as you progress."

☐ **Selects bag and connects to oxygen source capable of delivering 90% to 100% oxygen**

☐ **Selects appropriate-sized mask**

☐ **Tests bag**
  • **Good pressure?**   • **Pressure-release valve working?**   • **Valve assembly present and functioning?**
  • **Pressure manometer (if any) working? (If bag is not working properly, obtains and tests another)**

"The baby has just been born, placed under the radiant warmer, positioned, suctioned, dried, and given tactile stimulation. The baby is still apneic. Demonstrate what you would do for this baby."

☐ **Positions him/herself at the head or side of the baby and positions baby's head in "sniffing" position**

☐ **Positions bag and mask properly on baby**

☐ **Checks seal (gives two or three ventilations at appropriate pressure and observes for chest movement)**

"Rise"   "No Rise"

☐ **Checks for inadequate seal; repositions head and reapplies face mask**

"Yes" ◇ Rise

"No"

☐ **Checks for blocked airway**
  • **Repositions head**
  • **Checks for and removes secretions**
  • **Ventilates with mouth slightly open**

"Yes" ◇ Rise

"No"

☐ **Considers insufficient pressure**
  • **Increases ventilation pressure**
  • **Considers endotracheal intubation**

☐ **Ventilates for 30 seconds**
  • Rate: 40 to 60 times per minute
  • Pressure: Visible rise and fall of chest attained

☐ **Checks heart rate with stethoscope or umbilical palpation for 6 seconds***

| "Less than 6 beats" (<60 bpm) | "6 to 10 beats" (60 to 100 bpm) | "More than 10 beats" (>100 bpm) |

"Less than 6 beats"
(<60 bpm)

"6 to 10 beats"
(60 to 100 bpm)

"More than 10 beats"
(>100 bpm)

☐ **Continues ventilation**

☐ **Initiates chest compressions**

☐ **Considers intubation**

☐ **Continues ventilation**

☐ **Considers intubation**

☐ **Checks for spontaneous respirations**

"No spontaneous respirations"

"Yes, there are spontaneous respirations"

☐ **Continues positive-pressure ventilation**

☐ **Considers intubation and/or orogastric tube for prolonged ventilation**

☐ **Indicates need for ongoing care**

☐ **Gradually discontinues positive-pressure ventilation**

☐ **Provides tactile stimulation and free-flow oxygen**

☐ **Indicates need for ongoing care**

Instructor should present each of the scenarios separately and evaluate the learner's response for each.

☐ Correctly calculated baby's heart rate from 6-second count.

☐ Speed — no undue delays.

☐ Handling of baby was safe, with no trauma produced.

☐ Ventilated at appropriate rate (40 to 60 breaths per minute).

☐ Ventilated with appropriate pressure.

☐ Avoided using excessive pressure on mask.

☐ If ventilation continued longer than several minutes, an orogastric tube was inserted.

Key Points

1. Ventilation of the lungs is the single most important and most effective step in cardiopulmonary resuscitation of the compromised infant.

2. Indications for positive-pressure ventilation are
   - Apnea/gasping
   - Heart rate less than 100 beats per minute even if breathing
   - Persistent central cyanosis despite 100% free-flow oxygen

3. Preterm newborns are more likely to require assisted ventilation and endotracheal intubation than term infants.

4. Flow-inflating bags
   - Fill only when oxygen from a compressed source flows into them
   - Depend on a compressed gas source
   - Must have a tight face-mask seal to inflate
   - Use a flow-control valve to regulate pressure/inflation
   - Look like a deflated balloon when not in use

5. Self-inflating bags
   - Fill spontaneously after they are squeezed, pulling oxygen or air into the bag
   - Remain inflated at all times
   - Can deliver positive-pressure ventilation without a compressed gas source; user must be certain the bag is connected to an oxygen source for the purpose of neonatal resuscitation
   - Require attachment of an oxygen reservoir to deliver 100% oxygen

6. The flow-inflating bag will not work if
   - The mask is not properly sealed over the newborn's nose and mouth.
   - There is a tear in the bag.
   - The flow-control valve is open too wide.
   - The pressure gauge is missing.

7. Every resuscitation bag must have
   - A pressure release ("pop-off") valve
   and/or
   - A pressure gauge manometer and a flow-control valve

8. The self-inflating bag must have a reservoir; without the reservoir the bag delivers only about 40% oxygen, which is insufficient for neonatal resuscitation.

Key Points — *continued*

9. Corrective actions for no chest rise during bag-and-mask ventilation are

    • Reapply mask to face using light downward pressure.

    • Reposition the head.

    • Check for secretions, suction mouth and nose.

    • Ventilate with mouth slightly open.

    • Increase pressure of ventilations.

    • Recheck or replace the resuscitation bag.

    • After reasonable attempts fail, intubate the baby.

10. Improvement during bag-and-mask ventilation is indicated by

    • Increasing heart rate

    • Improving color

    • Spontaneous breathing

Answers to Questions

1. Flow-inflating bags **will not** work without a compressed gas source.

2. The next step is to **begin positive-pressure ventilation**.

3. **Ventilating the lungs** is the most important and effective step in neonatal resuscitation.

4. A. **flow-inflating**; B. **self-inflating**

5. Neonatal ventilation bags are **much smaller than** adult ventilation bags.

6. Self-inflating bags require the attachment of an **oxygen reservoir** to deliver 100% oxygen.

7. Masks of different sizes **do** need to be at every delivery.

Flow-inflating

8. Flow-inflating bags may fail to ventilate the baby because of (1) **inadequate seal between the mask and the face**, (2) **tear in the bag**, (3) **flow-control valve open too far**, and/or (4) **pressure manometer not attached or oxygen tubing disconnected or occluded**.

9. Illustration **C** is correct.

10. Pressure may be regulated by adjusting either the flowmeter or the **flow-control valve**.

Self-inflating

11. For a self-inflating bag to work, either the pressure manometer must be connected or the connection site must be **plugged**.

12. A self-inflating bag can deliver 90% to 100% oxygen **only when an oxygen reservoir is attached to it**.

13. Without an oxygen reservoir, a self-inflating bag can deliver only about **40%** oxygen.

14. The pressure delivered from a self-inflating bag is determined by (1) **how hard you squeeze the bag**, (2) **any leak that may be present between the mask and the baby's face**, and (3) **the set-point of the pressure-release valve**.

15. Free-flow oxygen can be delivered reliably only with a **flow-inflating bag**.

16. When giving free-flow oxygen, place the mask **loosely** on the baby's face to allow some gas to escape around the edges of the mask.

17. Mask **A** is correct.

18. The ventilation bag should be connected to **an oxygen source**.

19. When testing a resuscitation bag, you **make** an airtight seal between the mask and your palm.

20. When you test a flow-inflating bag, you watch to see if the bag **inflates**.

Answers to Questions — *continued*

21. When you squeeze the bag you **should** feel pressure against your hand.

22. The pressure manometer should read **30 to 40 cm H$_2$O**.

23. Baby **A** is positioned correctly.

24. Illustrations **A and B** are correct.

25. You should be able to see the newborn's **chest** and **abdomen**.

26. An anatomically shaped mask should be positioned with the **pointed** end over the newborn's nose.

27. If the chest is not rising, there may be (1) **an inadequate seal between the mask and face,** (2) **a blocked airway,** or (3) **insufficient pressure.**

28. You are **overinflating** the lungs, and there is danger you will produce a pneumothorax.

29. Squeeze the resuscitation bag at a rate of **40** to **60** breaths per minute.

30. Insert an **endotracheal tube** and begin bag-and-**tube** ventilation.

31. Use a **stethoscope** to listen for **breath** sounds in both lungs.

32. **Decrease** the rate and check the (1) **heart rate,** (2) **color,** and (3) **breathing.**

33. An **orogastric tube** should be inserted to act as a vent for the gas in the stomach.

34. The orogastric catheter should be inserted **22** cm (10 cm + 12 cm).

35. The syringe is removed, and the catheter is left **open** to vent stomach gas.

36. Bag-and-mask ventilation **should** continue.

37. The vast majority of babies requiring resuscitation **will** improve with positive-pressure ventilation by bag and mask.

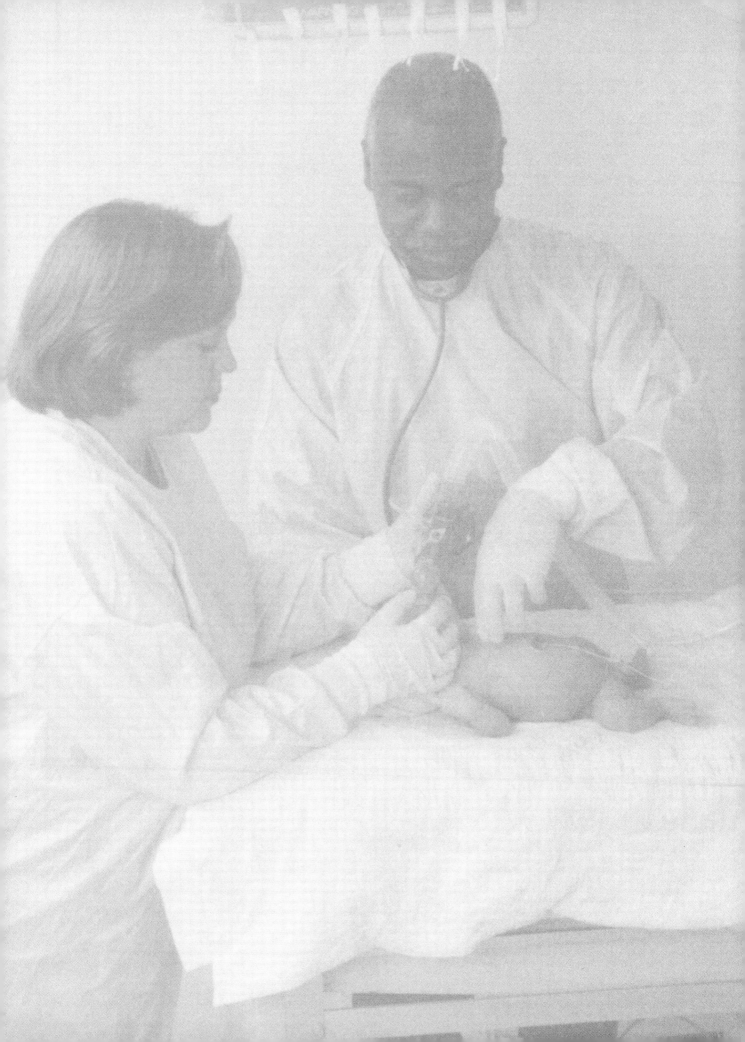

Chest Compressions

In Lesson 4 you will learn

- When to begin chest compressions during a resuscitation
- How to administer chest compressions
- How to coordinate chest compressions with positive-pressure ventilation
- When to stop chest compressions

The following case is an example of how chest compressions are delivered during a more extensive resuscitation. As you read the case, imagine yourself as part of the resuscitation team. The details of this step will be described in the remainder of the lesson.

Case 4. Resuscitation with positive-pressure ventilation and chest compressions

A pregnant woman contacts her obstetrician after noticing a pronounced decrease in fetal movements at 34 weeks' gestation.

Persistent fetal bradycardia is noted. Additional skilled personnel are called to the delivery room, the radiant warmer is turned on, and resuscitation equipment is prepared. An emergency cesarean section is performed, and a limp, apneic baby is given to the neonatal team.

The team positions the baby's head, suctions his mouth and nose, removes the wet linen, and stimulates him with drying and flicking the soles of his feet. However, 30 seconds after birth the baby is still limp, cyanotic, and without spontaneous respirations.

The team gives him positive-pressure ventilation with a bag-and-mask device using 100% oxygen. A gentle rise and fall of the chest is noted. However, after 30 seconds of this, the baby has a very low heart rate (20 to 30 beats per minute [bpm]) and remains cyanotic and limp.

The team begins chest compressions coordinated with positive-pressure ventilation. Repeated assessments are made to be certain that the airway is clear and the head is positioned correctly. However, ventilation with the bag and mask is not adequately moving the chest and, after another 30 seconds, the heart rate has not increased.

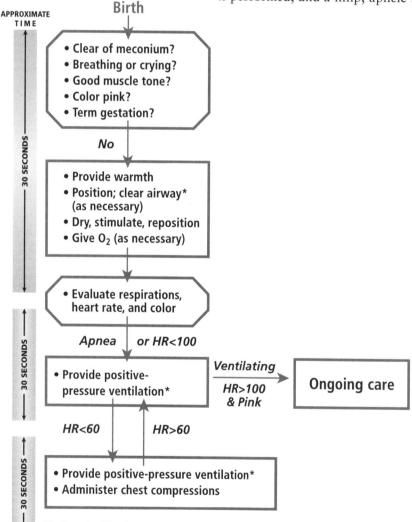

APPROXIMATE TIME

30 SECONDS

Birth

- Clear of meconium?
- Breathing or crying?
- Good muscle tone?
- Color pink?
- Term gestation?

No

- Provide warmth
- Position; clear airway* (as necessary)
- Dry, stimulate, reposition
- Give O₂ (as necessary)

- Evaluate respirations, heart rate, and color

Apnea or *HR<100*

30 SECONDS

- Provide positive-pressure ventilation*

Ventilating
HR>100 & Pink

Ongoing care

HR<60   *HR>60*

30 SECONDS

- Provide positive-pressure ventilation*
- Administer chest compressions

*Endotracheal intubation may be considered at several steps.

The trachea is rapidly intubated to ensure effective ventilation, and coordinated chest compressions and positive-pressure ventilation are resumed. Positive-pressure ventilation now appears to be resulting in better chest movement.

The baby finally makes an initial gasp. Chest compressions are stopped when the heart rate is noted to rise above 60 bpm. The team continues assisted ventilation with 100% oxygen, and stimulation is provided by rubbing the baby's back. His color improves, and the heart rate rises to more than 100 bpm. After he shows some spontaneous respirations, he is moved to the nursery for careful monitoring and further management.

What will this lesson cover?

Your first 30 seconds of resuscitating this baby were spent clearing his airway by positioning, suctioning, drying him, and using other forms of stimulation to encourage him to breathe. You checked the heart rate and found it to be less than 100 bpm. There were no spontaneous respirations. You then administered effective positive-pressure ventilation (as determined by good chest movement and breath sounds) with 100% oxygen for another 30 seconds and checked the heart rate again.

By this time, the vast majority of babies who require resuscitation will have shown some improvement as a result of improved ventilation. A few will remain apneic with a heart rate less than 60 bpm. These babies should receive chest compressions, coordinated with continuing positive-pressure ventilation. During this process, endotracheal intubation may be indicated to ensure effective ventilation.

This lesson will teach the technique of administering chest compressions. Endotracheal intubation is taught in Lesson 5.

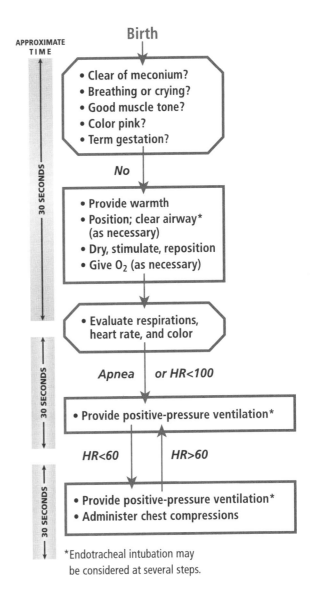

What are the indications for beginning chest compressions?

 Chest compressions should be started whenever the heart rate remains less than 60 bpm despite 30 seconds of effective positive-pressure ventilation.

Why perform chest compressions?

Babies who have a heart rate below 60 bpm, despite stimulation and 30 seconds of positive-pressure ventilation, probably have very low blood oxygen levels. As a result, the myocardium is depressed and unable to contract strongly enough to pump blood to the lungs to pick up the oxygen that you have now ensured is in the lungs. Therefore, you will need to mechanically pump the heart while you simultaneously continue to ventilate the lungs with 100% oxygen until the myocardium becomes sufficiently oxygenated to recover adequate spontaneous function. This process also will help to restore oxygen delivery to the brain.

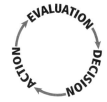 Those who are skilled at endotracheal intubation may choose to intubate at this time to ensure that ventilation is adequate and to facilitate the coordination of ventilation and chest compressions.

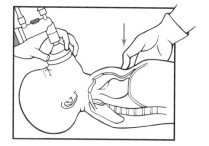

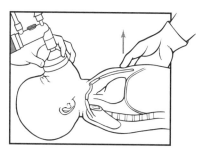

Figure 4.1. Compression (top) and release (bottom) phases of chest compressions

What are chest compressions?

Chest compressions, sometimes referred to as *external cardiac massage*, consist of rhythmic compressions of the sternum that

• Compress the heart against the spine.

• Increase the intrathoracic pressure.

• Circulate blood to the vital organs of the body.

The heart lies in the chest between the lower third of the sternum and the spine. Compressing the sternum compresses the heart and increases the pressure in the chest, causing blood to be pumped into the arteries (Figure 4.1).

When pressure on the sternum is released, blood enters the heart from the veins.

How many people are needed to administer chest compressions, and where should they stand?

Remember that chest compressions are of little value unless the lungs are also being ventilated with oxygen. Therefore, two people are required to administer chest compressions — one to compress the chest and one to continue ventilation.

As you will learn, these two people will need to coordinate their activities, so it will be helpful if both of them practice beforehand. The person performing chest compressions must have access to the chest and be able to position his or her hands correctly. The person assisting ventilation will need to be positioned at the baby's head to achieve an effective mask-face seal (or to stabilize the endotracheal tube) and watch for effective chest rise (Figure 4.2).

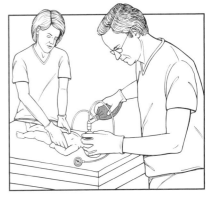

Figure 4.2. Two people are required when chest compressions are given.

How do you position your hands on the chest to begin chest compressions?

You will learn two different techniques for performing chest compressions. These techniques are

- Thumb technique
- Two-finger technique

Each technique has advantages and disadvantages. Based on a limited amount of data, the thumb technique is preferred, but the two-finger technique is acceptable.

With the thumb technique, the two thumbs are used to depress the sternum, while the hands encircle the torso and the fingers support the spine (Figure 4.3A). If the baby is large and your hands are small, you should be sure that the baby is on a firm surface.

With the two-finger technique, the tips of the middle finger and either the index finger or ring finger of one hand are used to compress the sternum. The other hand is used to support the baby's back, unless the baby is on a very firm surface (Figure 4.3B).

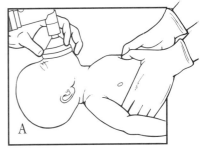

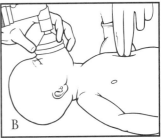

Figure 4.3. Two techniques for giving chest compressions: thumb (A) and two-finger (B)

What are the advantages of one technique over the other?

The thumb technique is preferred because it is usually less tiring, and you can generally control the depth of compression somewhat better. It also is preferable for individuals with long fingernails. However, the two-finger technique is more convenient if the baby is large or your hands are small. The two-finger technique also is preferable to provide access to the umbilicus when medications need to be given by the umbilical route. Therefore, you should learn both techniques.

The two techniques have the following things in common:

• Position of the baby
  – Firm support for the back
  – Neck slightly extended
• Compressions
  – Same location, depth, and rate

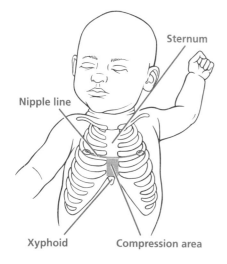

Figure 4.4. Landmarks for chest compressions

Where on the chest should you position your thumbs or fingers?

When chest compressions are performed on a newborn, pressure is applied to the lower third of the sternum, which lies between the xyphoid and a line drawn between the nipples (Figure 4.4). The xyphoid is the small projection where the lower ribs meet at the midline. You can quickly locate the correct area on the sternum by running your fingers along the lower edge of the ribs until you locate the xyphoid. Then place your thumbs or fingers immediately above the xyphoid. Care must be used to avoid putting pressure directly on the xyphoid.

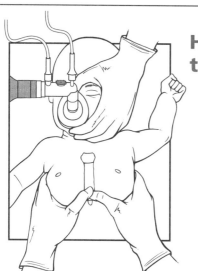
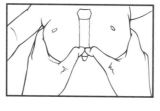

How do you position your hands using the thumb technique?

The thumb technique is accomplished by encircling the torso with both hands and placing the thumbs on the sternum and the fingers under the newborn.

The thumbs can be placed side by side or, on a small baby, one over the other (Figure 4.5).

Figure 4.5. Thumb technique of chest compressions for small (left) and large (right) babies

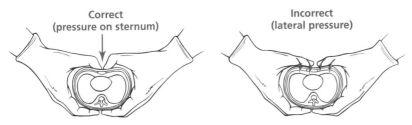

Figure 4.6. Correct and incorrect application of pressure with thumb technique of chest compressions

The thumbs will be used to compress the sternum, while your fingers provide the support needed for the back. The thumbs should be flexed at the first joint and pressure applied vertically to compress the heart between the sternum and the spine (Figure 4.6).

The thumb technique has some restrictions. It cannot be used effectively if the baby is large or your hands are small. It also makes access to the umbilical cord more difficult when medications become necessary.

How do you position your hands using the two-finger technique?

In the two-finger technique, the tips of your middle finger and either the index or ring finger of one hand are used for compressions (Figure 4.7). You will probably find it easier to use your right hand if you are right-handed, your left hand if you are left-handed. Position the two fingers perpendicular to the chest as shown, and press with your fingertips. If you find that your nails prevent you from using your fingertips, you should ventilate the newborn while your partner compresses the chest. Alternatively, you could use the thumb technique for performing chest compressions.

Your other hand should be used to support the newborn's back so that the heart is more effectively compressed between the sternum and spine. With the second hand supporting the back, you can feel the pressure and the depth of compressions.

When compressing the chest, only the two fingertips should rest on the chest. This way, you can best control the pressure you apply to the sternum and the spine (Figure 4.8A).

As with the thumb technique, you should apply pressure vertically to compress the heart between the sternum and the spine. (Figure 4.8A).

You may find the two-finger technique to be more tiring than the thumb technique if chest compressions are required for a prolonged period. However, the two-finger technique can be used regardless of the size of the baby or the size of your hands. An additional advantage of this technique is that it leaves the umbilicus more accessible in case medications must be administered via the umbilical route.

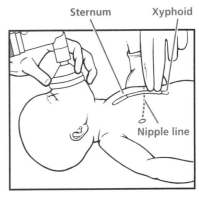

Figure 4.7. Correct finger position for chest compressions

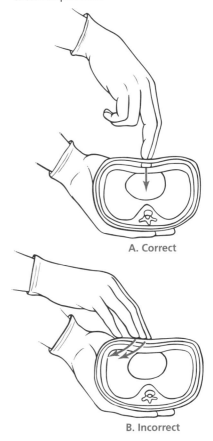

A. Correct

B. Incorrect

Figure 4.8. Correct and incorrect application of pressure with two-finger technique

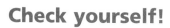

Check yourself!

(The answers are in the preceding section and at the end of the lesson.)

1. A newborn is apneic and blue. Her airway is cleared, and she is stimulated. At 30 seconds, positive-pressure ventilation is begun. At 60 seconds, her heart rate is 80 beats per minute. Chest compressions (should) (should not) be started. Positive-pressure ventilation (should) (should not) be continued.

2. A newborn is apneic and blue. She remains apneic despite having her airway cleared, being stimulated, and receiving 30 seconds of positive-pressure ventilation. At 60 seconds, her heart rate is 40 beats per minute. Chest compressions (should) (should not) be started. Positive-pressure ventilation (should) (should not) be continued.

3. During the compression phase of chest compressions, the sternum compresses the heart, which causes blood to be pumped from the heart into the (veins) (arteries). In the release phase, blood enters the heart from the (veins) (arteries).

4. Mark the area on this baby where you would apply chest compressions.

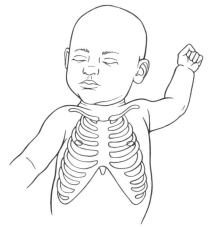

5. The preferred method of delivering chest compressions is the (thumb) (two-finger) technique.

6. If you anticipate that the baby will need medication by the umbilical route, it may be easier to deliver chest compressions with the (thumb) (two-finger) technique.

How much pressure do you use to compress the chest?

Controlling the pressure used in compressing the sternum is an important part of the procedure.

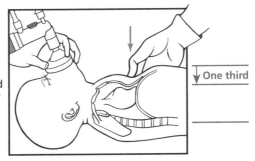

Figure 4.9. Compression depth should be approximately one third of the anterior-posterior diameter of the chest.

One third

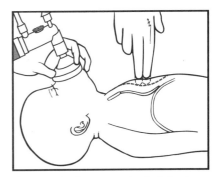

Figure 4.10. *Correct* method of chest compressions (fingers remain in contact with chest on release)

With your fingers and hands correctly positioned, you should use enough pressure to depress the sternum *to a depth of approximately one third of the anterior-posterior diameter of the chest,* then release the pressure to allow the heart to refill (Figure 4.9). One compression consists of the downward stroke plus the release. The actual distance compressed will depend on the size of the baby.

The duration of the downward stroke of the compression should also be somewhat shorter than the duration of the release for generation of maximum cardiac output.

Your thumbs or the tips of your fingers (depending on the method you use) should remain in contact with the chest at all times during both compression *and* release (Figure 4.10). *Do not* lift your thumbs or fingers off the chest between compressions (Figure 4.11). If you take your thumbs or fingers completely off the sternum after compression, then

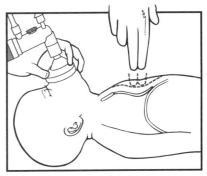

Figure 4.11. *Incorrect* method of chest compressions (fingers lose contact with chest on release)

- You waste time relocating the compression area.
- You lose control over the depth of compression.
- You may compress the wrong area, producing trauma to the chest or underlying organs.

Are there dangers associated with administering chest compressions?

Chest compressions can cause trauma to the baby.

Two vital organs lie within the ribcage — the heart and lungs. The liver lies partially under the ribs, although it is in the abdominal cavity. As you perform chest compressions, you must apply enough pressure to compress the heart between the sternum and spine without damaging underlying organs. Pressure applied too low, over the xyphoid, can cause laceration of the liver (Figure 4.12).

Also, the ribs are fragile and can easily be broken.

By following the procedure outlined in this lesson, the risk of these injuries can be minimized.

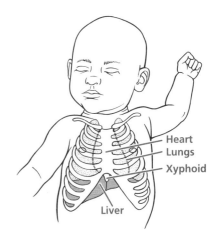

Heart
Lungs
Xyphoid

Liver

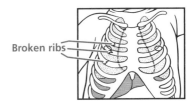

Broken ribs

Figure 4.12. Structures that may be damaged during chest compressions

How often do you compress the chest and coordinate with ventilation?

During cardiopulmonary resuscitation, chest compressions must always be accompanied by positive-pressure ventilation. But you should avoid giving a compression and a ventilation simultaneously, since one will decrease the efficacy of the other. Therefore, the two activities must be coordinated, with one ventilation interposed after every third compression, for a total of 30 breaths and 90 compressions per minute (Figure 4.13).

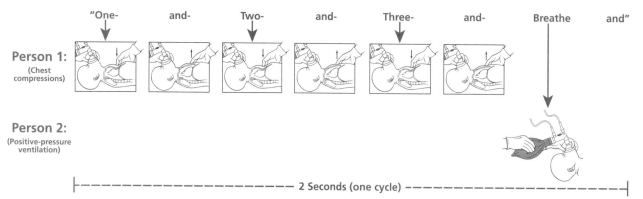

Figure 4.13. Coordination of chest compressions and ventilation

The person doing the compressions should take over the counting out loud from the person who is doing the ventilating. The compressor should count "One-and-Two-and-Three-and-Breathe-and" while the person ventilating squeezes during "Breathe-and" and releases during "One-and." Note that passive exhalation occurs during the downward stroke of the next compression. Counting the cadence will help develop a smooth and well-coordinated procedure.

One *cycle of events* will consist of three compressions plus one ventilation.

• A four-event cycle should take approximately 2 seconds.

• There should be approximately 120 "events" per minute (90 compressions plus 30 breaths).

Note that during chest compressions the ventilation rate is actually 30 breaths per minute rather than the rate you previously learned for positive-pressure ventilation, which was 40 to 60 breaths per minute. This lower ventilatory rate is needed to provide an adequate number of compressions and avoid simultaneous compressions and ventilation. To ensure that the process can be coordinated, it is important for you to practice with another person and to practice the roles of both the compressor and the ventilator.

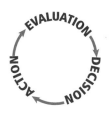

While chest compressions and positive-pressure ventilation are being delivered, there is a higher likelihood that air will enter the stomach. Therefore, unless you have already done so, it now would be advisable to pass an orogastric tube to vent the stomach. Also, many will have inserted an endotracheal tube by this time to reduce the chances of stomach inflation and to improve the efficacy of ventilation.

How can you practice the rhythm of chest compressions with ventilation?

Imagine that you are the person giving chest compressions. Repeat the words several times while you move your hand to compress the chest on "One-and," "Two-and," "Three-and." Do not press when you say, "Breathe-and." Do not remove your fingers from the surface you are pressing.

Now time yourself to see if you can say and do these five cycles of events in 10 seconds. Remember not to press on the "Breathe-and."

Practice saying the words and compressing the chest.

One-and-Two-and-Three-and-Breathe-and-One-and-Two-and-Three-and-Breathe-and-One-and-Two-and-Three-and-Breathe-and-One-and-Two-and-Three-and-Breathe-and-One-and-Two-and-Three-and-Breathe-and

Now imagine that you are the person administering bag-and-mask ventilation. This time you want to squeeze your hand when you say "Breathe-and" but not when you say "One-and," "Two-and," "Three-and."

Now time yourself to see if you can say and do these five events in 10 seconds. Remember, squeeze your hand only when you say "Breathe-and."

*One-and-Two-and-Three-and-**Breathe-and**-One-and-Two-and-Three-and-**Breathe-and**-One-and-Two-and-Three-and-**Breathe-and**-One-and-Two-and-Three-and-**Breathe-and**-One-and-Two-and-Three-and-**Breathe-and***

In a real situation, there will be two resuscitators, with one doing the compressions and one doing the bagging. The person compressing will be speaking "One-and-Two-and- ..." out loud. Therefore, it will be helpful for you to practice with a partner, taking turns in each of the roles.

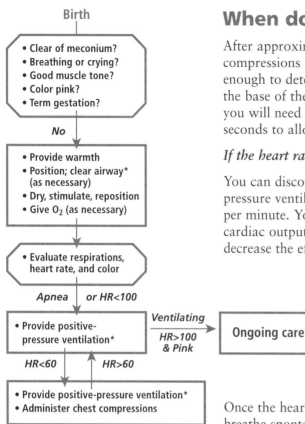

*Endotracheal intubation may
be considered at several steps.

When do you stop chest compressions?

After approximately 30 seconds of well-coordinated chest compressions and ventilation, you should stop compressions long enough to determine the heart rate again. If you can feel the pulse at the base of the cord, you will not need to stop ventilation. Otherwise, you will need to stop both compressions and ventilation for a few seconds to allow you to listen to the chest with a stethoscope.

If the heart rate is now above 60 bpm, then

You can discontinue chest compressions, but continue positive-pressure ventilation now at the more rapid rate of 40 to 60 breaths per minute. You should not continue chest compressions, since the cardiac output is probably adequate and the compressions may decrease the effectiveness of the positive-pressure ventilation.

Once the heart rate rises above 100 bpm and the baby begins to breathe spontaneously, you should slowly withdraw positive-pressure ventilation, as described in Lesson 3, and move the baby to the nursery for ongoing care.

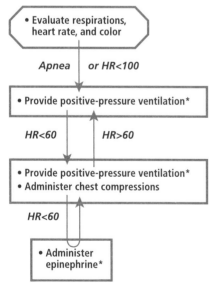

*Endotracheal intubation may
be considered at several steps.

What do you do if the baby is not improving?

While you are administering chest compressions and coordinated ventilation, you should continue to ask yourself the following questions:

- Is chest movement adequate? (Have you considered or performed endotracheal intubation?)
- Is 100% oxygen being given?
- Is the depth of chest compression approximately one third of the diameter of the chest?
- Are the chest compressions and ventilation being well coordinated?

If the heart rate remains below 60 bpm, then you should give epinephrine, as described in Lesson 6.

As discussed previously, by this point in a resuscitation you most likely will have intubated the trachea. In addition to giving you a more reliable means of ventilating the baby (particularly when coordinating ventilation and chest compressions), the endotracheal tube provides a route for administering epinephrine. The technique of endotracheal intubation will be described in Lesson 5, and a description of administering epinephrine appears in Lesson 6.

Lesson 4 Review

(The answers are at the end of the lesson.)

1. A newborn is apneic and blue. Her airway is cleared, and she is stimulated. At 30 seconds, positive-pressure ventilation is begun. At 60 seconds, her heart rate is 80 beats per minute. Chest compressions (should) (should not) be started. Positive-pressure ventilation (should) (should not) be continued.

2. A newborn is apneic and blue. She remains apneic despite having her airway cleared, being stimulated, and receiving 30 seconds of positive-pressure ventilation. At 60 seconds, her heart rate is 40 beats per minute. Chest compressions (should) (should not) be started. Positive-pressure ventilation (should) (should not) be continued.

3. During the compression phase of chest compressions, the sternum compresses the heart, which causes blood to be pumped from the heart into the (veins) (arteries). In the release phase, blood enters the heart from the (veins) (arteries).

4. Mark the area on this baby where you would apply chest compressions.

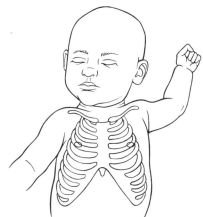

5. The preferred method of delivering chest compressions is the (thumb) (two-finger) technique.

6. If you anticipate that the baby will need medication by the umbilical route, it may be easier to deliver chest compressions with the (thumb) (two-finger) technique.

Lesson 4 Review — *continued*

(The answers are at the end of the lesson.)

7. The correct depth of chest compressions is approximately

   A. One fourth of the anterior-posterior diameter of the chest

   B. One third of the anterior-posterior diameter of the chest

   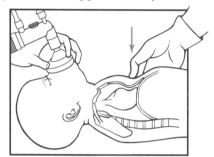

   C. One half of the anterior-posterior diameter of the chest

8. Which drawing shows the correct release motion?

   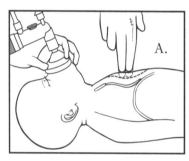 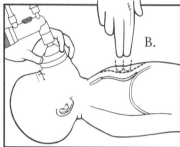

9. What phrase is used to time and coordinate chest compressions and ventilation? _____.

10. The ratio of chest compressions to ventilation is _____ to _____.

11. During positive-pressure ventilation without chest compressions, the rate of breaths per minute should be _____ to _____ breaths per minute.

12. During positive-pressure ventilation with chest compressions, the rate of "events" per minute should be _____ "events" per minute.

Lesson 4 Review — *continued*

(The answers are at the end of the lesson.)

13. The count "One-and-Two-and-Three-and-Breathe-and" should take about _____ seconds.

14. A baby has required ventilation and chest compressions. After 30 seconds of chest compressions, you stop and count **eight heartbeats in 6 seconds.** The baby's heart rate is now _____ beats per minute. You should (continue) (stop) chest compressions.

15. A baby has required chest compressions and is being ventilated with bag and mask. The chest is not moving well. You stop and count **four heartbeats in 6 seconds.** The baby's heart rate is now _____ beats per minute. You may want to consider

    _____   _____.

16. Complete the chart.

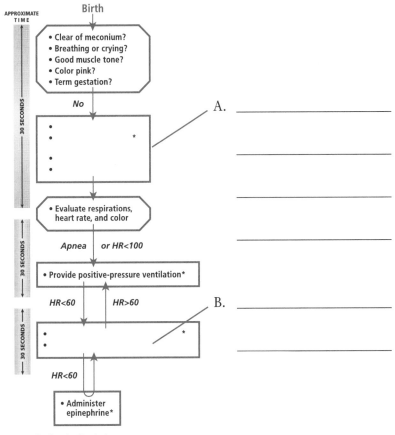

APPROXIMATE TIME

Birth

• Clear of meconium?
• Breathing or crying?
• Good muscle tone?
• Color pink?
• Term gestation?

No

30 SECONDS

*

A. _____

_____

_____

_____

• Evaluate respirations, heart rate, and color

Apnea or *HR<100*

30 SECONDS

• Provide positive-pressure ventilation*

HR<60   *HR>60*

B. _____

_____

30 SECONDS

•
•

*

HR<60

• Administer epinephrine*

*Endotracheal intubation may be considered at several steps.

Performance Checklist
Lesson 4 — Chest Compressions

Instructor: The learner should be instructed to talk through the procedure as it is demonstrated. Judge the performance of each step and check (✓) the box when the action is completed correctly. If done incorrectly, circle the box so that you can discuss that step later. At several points, you will need to provide information concerning the condition of the baby.

Learner: To successfully complete this checklist, you should be able to perform all the steps and make all the correct decisions in the procedure. You should talk through the procedure as you perform it.

Equipment and Supplies
Newborn resuscitation manikin

Radiant warmer or table to simulate warmer

Gloves (or may be implied)

Stethoscope

Self-inflating bag

     or

Flow-inflating bag with pressure manometer and oxygen source

Clock with second hand

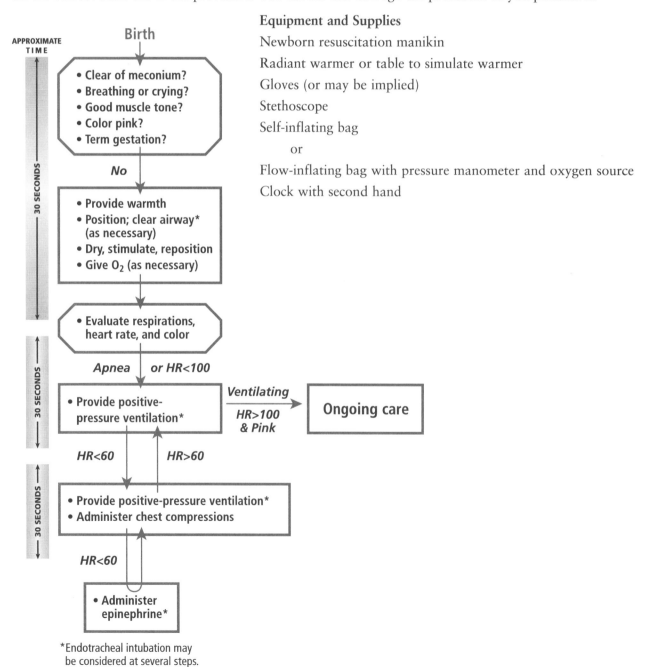

*Endotracheal intubation may be considered at several steps.

Continued on page 4-17

Neonatal Resuscitation

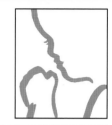

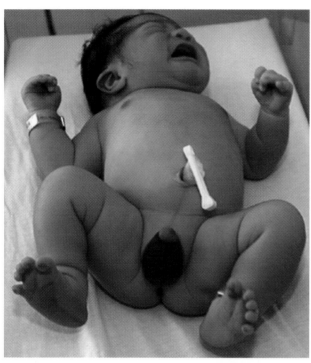

Fig A-1. Normal newborn. Good color and good tone are present. Note absence of central cyanosis and presence of pink color of mucous membranes. Supplemental oxygen is not needed.

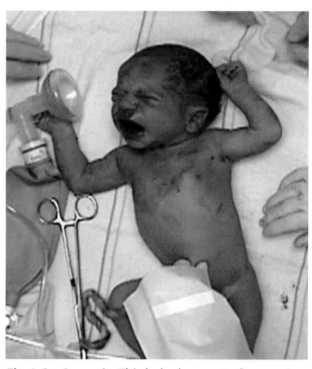

Fig A-2. Cyanosis. This baby has central cyanosis. Supplemental oxygen and perhaps assisted ventilation are needed.

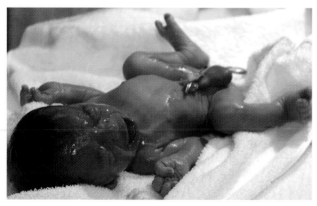

Fig A-3. Newborn immediately following birth. Drying and removing the wet linen will probably stimulate breathing and prevent body cooling.

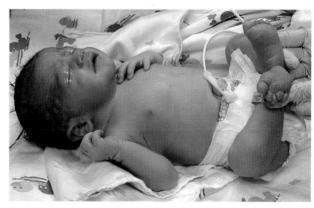

Fig A-4. Acrocyanosis. This baby has acrocyanosis of hands and feet, but trunk and mucous membranes are pink. Supplemental oxygen is not required.

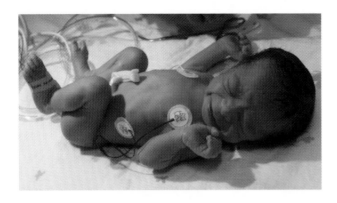

Fig. B-1. At-risk newborn: good tone. This baby is slightly preterm and small for gestational age. However, tone is excellent.

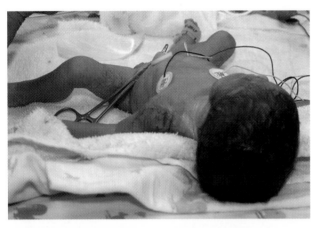

Fig. B-2. At-risk newborn: poor tone. This baby's poor tone is worse than one would anticipate simply from her being born preterm. Resuscitation is required.

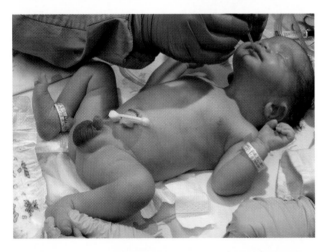

Fig. B-3. At-risk newborn: pale. This baby is very pale and there was a history of placenta previa. Volume expansion may be required.

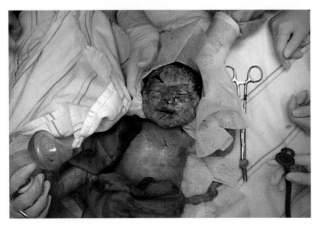

Fig. B-4. At-risk newborn: meconium. This newborn is covered with meconium and is not vigorous (poor tone and poor respiratory effort). Endotracheal intubation and suctioning are required.

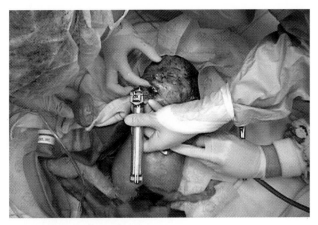

Fig C-1a. Limp baby covered with meconium. Resuscitator is preparing to perform endotracheal intubation and suctioning.

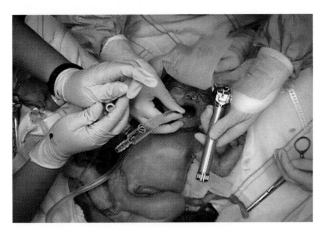

Fig. C-1b. An endotracheal tube has been inserted, a meconium aspiration device has been connected to the tube, and the suction tubing is about to be connected.

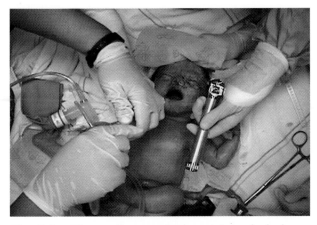

Fig. C-1c. The suction control port is occluded so that the suction is applied to the endotracheal tube as the tube is gradually withdrawn.

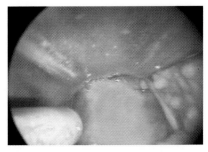

Fig. C-2a. View of posterior pharynx after first inserting laryngoscope

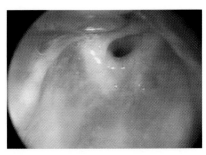

Fig. C-2b. View of esophagus after laryngoscope has been inserted slightly too far

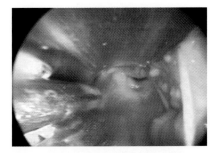

Fig. C-2c. View of arytenoids and posterior glottis as laryngoscope blade is withdrawn slightly

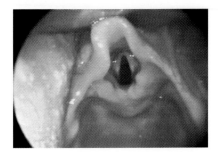

Fig. C-2d. View of glottis and vocal cords as laryngoscope is gently lifted

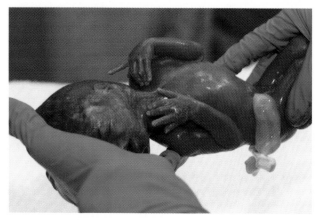

Fig. D-1. This extremely preterm baby is cyanotic, has poor muscle tone, and requires assisted ventilation.

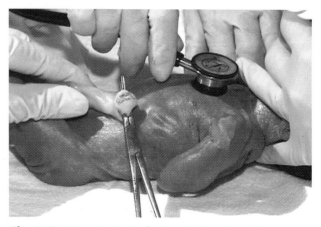

Fig. D-2. Heart rate is being determined by two methods: palpating the base of the cord and listening to the chest.

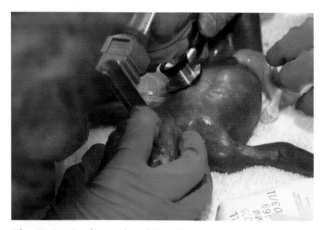

Fig. D-3. Endotracheal intubation procedure is begun as assistant listens to the heart rate.

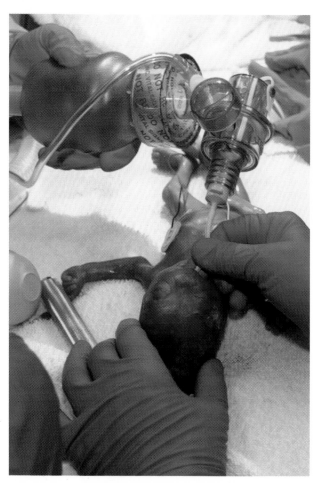

Fig. D-4. Endotracheal tube is held in place as positive pressure ventilation is provided.

Performance Checklist
Lesson 4 — Chest Compressions

Name _____ Instructor _____ Date _____

This performance checklist includes responsibilities for two learners: one who ventilates the baby and one who provides chest compressions. If only one learner is being evaluated, the instructor should assume the role of the other learner. The location of the check box indicates which learner is responsible for each activity. Each learner should demonstrate skills in both roles, and each learner must serve as Learner #1 twice to demonstrate both methods of performing chest compressions.

Instructor's questions are in quotes. Learner's questions and correct responses are in bold type. Instructor should check boxes as the learner answers correctly.

"This baby born at term has been provided warmth, positioned, suctioned, dried, and given tactile stimulation. He remains apneic."

Learner #1   **Learner #2**

Initiates bag-and-mask ventilation with 100% oxygen   ☐

After 30 seconds, asks for heart rate check   ☐

☐ **Checks the heart rate by palpation for exactly 6 seconds**

"You detect four beats in 6 seconds."

☐ **Announces heart rate of 40 bpm and indicates need for chest compressions**

☐ **Locates appropriate position on lower one third of sternum**

☐ **Provides firm support for baby's back**

Two-finger technique   Thumb technique

☐ **Uses fingertips of middle**   ☐ **Uses distal portion of**
   and index or ring fingers   **both thumbs**

☐ **Compresses sternum approximately one third of the anterior-posterior diameter of chest**

☐ **Keeps fingertips/thumbs on sternum during release**

☐ **Brings tempo to approximately two compressions per second with a pause after every third compression for ventilation; counts cadence ("One-and-Two-and-Three-and-Breathe-and...")**

Learner #1   Learner #2

        Ventilates during the pause after every third compression   ☐

        **Provides adequate ventilation pressure and head/mask placement
to achieve adequate chest movement**   ☐

☐   **Checks the heart rate by palpation for exactly 6 seconds after 30 seconds of
chest compressions**

"You detect no pulsations."

☐   **Learner #2 ceases ventilation while Learner #1 checks the heart rate by auscultation**   ☐

"You detect five beats in 6 seconds."

☐   **Announces heart rate of 50 bpm and resumes chest compressions**

        Resumes ventilation immediately after heart rate check and considers   ☐

           • **Is chest movement adequate?**

           • **Is 100% oxygen being given?**

           • **Is the depth of chest compression approximately one third
the diameter of the chest?**

           • **Are chest compressions and ventilation being well coordinated?**

           • **Are endotracheal intubation and epinephrine indicated?**

☐   **Checks heart rate by palpation for exactly 6 seconds 30 seconds after previous
heart rate check**

"You detect nine beats in 6 seconds."

☐   **Announces heart rate of 90 bpm and discontinues chest compressions**

        Continues ventilation   ☐

Overall performance, judged after performing both roles

☐ Correctly coordinated chest compressions with ventilation

☐ Correctly stated whether chest compressions should be stopped or continued, depending on heart rate

☐ Correctly performed thumb technique

☐ Correctly performed two-finger technique

☐ Correctly evaluated heart rate at appropriate times (first palpated cord then, if necessary, ceased ventilation
and listened to chest with stethoscope)

☐ Speed — carried out action without undue delay

Key Points

1. Chest compressions are indicated when the heart rate remains less than 60 beats per minute despite 30 seconds of effective positive-pressure ventilation.

2. Chest compressions
   - Compress the heart against the spine.
   - Increase intrathoracic pressure.
   - Circulate blood to the vital organs, including the brain.

3. There are two acceptable techniques for chest compressions — the thumb technique and the two-finger technique, but the thumb technique is usually preferred.

4. Locate the correct area for compressions by running your fingers along the lower edge of the ribs until you locate the xyphoid. Then place your thumbs or fingers on the sternum, immediately above the xyphoid.

5. To ensure proper rate of chest compressions and ventilation, the compressor repeats "One-and-Two-and-Three-and-Breathe-and...."

6. During chest compressions, the breathing rate is 30 breaths per minute and the compression rate is 90 compressions per minute. This equals 120 "events" per minute. One cycle of three compressions and one breath takes 2 seconds.

7. During chest compressions, ensure that
   - Chest movement is adequate during ventilation.
   - 100% oxygen is being used.
   - Compression depth is one third the diameter of the chest.
   - Thumbs or fingers remain in contact with the chest at all times.
   - Duration of the downward stroke of the compression is shorter than duration of the release.
   - Chest compressions and ventilation are well coordinated.

8. After 30 seconds of chest compressions and ventilation, check the heart rate. If the heart rate is
   - Greater than 60 beats per minute, discontinue compressions and continue ventilation at 40 to 60 breaths per minute.
   - Greater than 100 beats per minute, discontinue compressions, and gradually discontinue ventilation if the newborn is breathing spontaneously.
   - Less than 60 beats per minute, intubate the newborn, if not already done. This provides a more reliable method of continuing ventilation and a route for epinephrine.

Answers to Questions

1. Chest compressions **should not** be started. Positive-pressure ventilation **should** be continued.

2. Chest compressions **should** be started. Positive-pressure ventilation **should** be continued.

3. Blood is pumped into the **arteries** during the compression phase and from the **veins** during the release phase.

4. Compression area

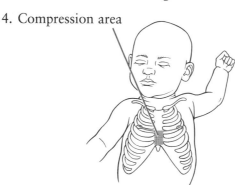

5. The preferred method of delivering chest compressions is the **thumb** technique.

6. The **two-finger** technique may be easier if medications will be given by the umbilical route.

7. The correct depth of chest compressions is approximately **one third of the anterior-posterior diameter of the chest** (B).

8. Drawing **A** is correct (fingers remain in contact during release).

9. **"One-and-Two-and-Three-and-Breathe-and ..."**

10. The ratio is **3:1.**

11. The rate of ventilation without chest compressions should be **40 to 60** breaths per minute.

12. There should be **120** "events" per minute during chest compressions.

13. The count "One-and-Two-and-Three-and-Breathe-and" should take about **2** seconds.

14. Eight heartbeats in 6 seconds is **80** beats per minute. You should **stop** chest compressions.

15. Four heartbeats in 6 seconds is **40** beats per minute. You may want to consider **endotracheal intubation.**

16. A.   B.

• Provide warmth • Position; clear airway   (as necessary) • Dry, stimulate, reposition • Give O₂ (as necessary)

• Provide positive-pressure ventilation • Administer chest compressions

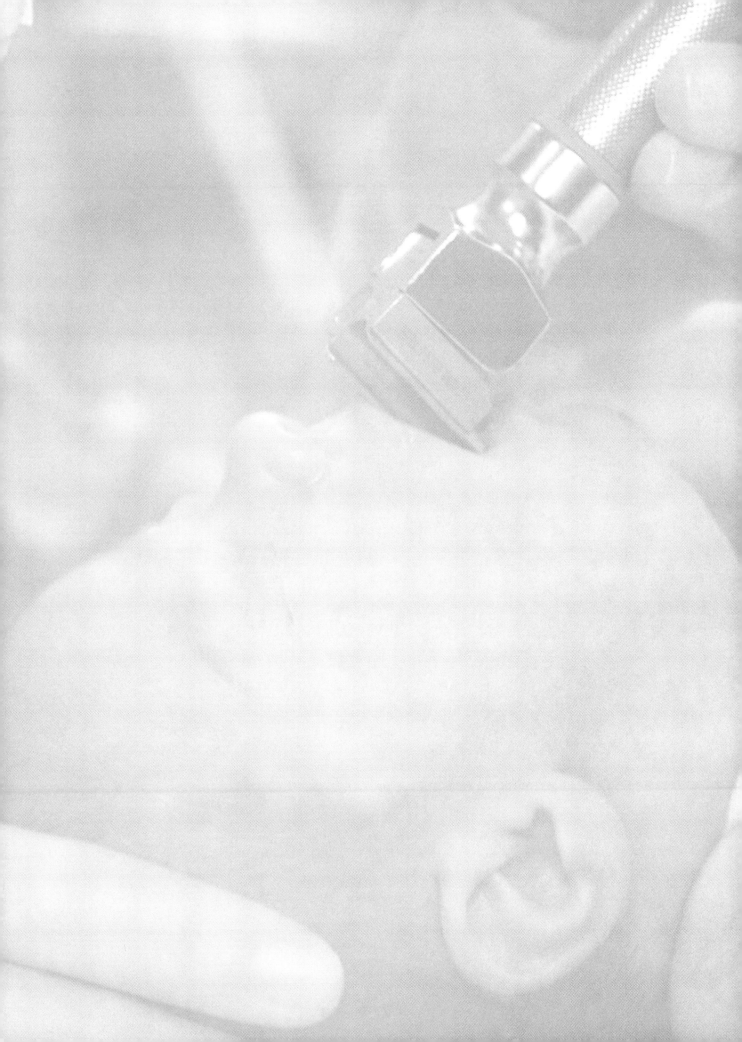

Endotracheal Intubation

In Lesson 5 you will learn

- When and why endotracheal intubation is needed during resuscitation
- How to prepare the equipment needed for endotracheal intubation
- How to use the laryngoscope to insert an endotracheal tube
- How to determine if the endotracheal tube is in the trachea
- How to use the endotracheal tube to suction meconium from the trachea
- How to use the endotracheal tube to administer positive-pressure ventilation

When is endotracheal intubation required?

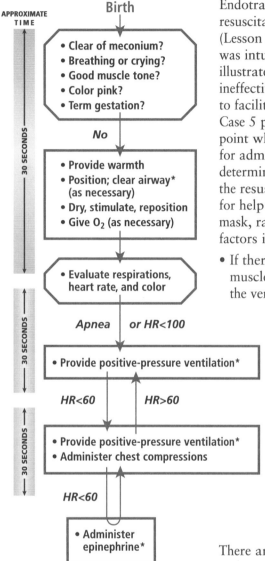

APPROXIMATE TIME

Birth

30 SECONDS

- Clear of meconium?
- Breathing or crying?
- Good muscle tone?
- Color pink?
- Term gestation?

No

- Provide warmth
- Position; clear airway* (as necessary)
- Dry, stimulate, reposition
- Give O₂ (as necessary)

- Evaluate respirations, heart rate, and color

Apnea or *HR<100*

30 SECONDS

- Provide positive-pressure ventilation*

HR<60 *HR>60*

30 SECONDS

- Provide positive-pressure ventilation*
- Administer chest compressions

HR<60

- Administer epinephrine*

*Endotracheal intubation may be considered at several steps.

Endotracheal intubation may be performed at various points during a resuscitation as indicated by the asterisks in the flow diagram. Case 2 (Lesson 2, page 2-3) illustrated one such point, where the trachea was intubated to suction meconium. Case 4 (Lesson 4, page 4-2) illustrated another point, where bag-and-mask ventilation was ineffective and the trachea was intubated to improve ventilation and to facilitate the coordinating of ventilation and chest compressions. Case 5 presented in Lesson 6 (page 6-2) will illustrate yet another point where endotracheal intubation is valuable — to provide a route for administering epinephrine. The timing of intubation will be determined by many factors, one of which is the intubation skill of the resuscitator. People who are not adept at intubation should call for help and focus on providing effective ventilation with bag and mask, rather than wasting valuable time trying to intubate. Other factors influencing the timing of intubation include the following:

- If there is meconium and the baby has depressed respirations, muscle tone, or heart rate, you will need to intubate the trachea as the very first step, before any other resuscitation measures are started.

  - If positive-pressure ventilation by bag and mask is not resulting in good chest rise, or if the need for positive-pressure ventilation lasts beyond a few minutes, you may decide to intubate simply to improve the efficacy and ease of assisted ventilation.

  - If chest compressions are necessary, intubating may facilitate coordination of chest compressions and ventilation and maximize the efficiency of each positive-pressure breath.

  - As you will learn in the next lesson, if epinephrine is required to stimulate the heart, one common route to administer the epinephrine is directly into the trachea. This too will require endotracheal intubation.

There are also some special indications for endotracheal intubation, such as for extreme prematurity, surfactant administration, and suspected diaphragmatic hernia. These indications will be discussed in Lesson 7.

Note: Masks that fit over the laryngeal inlet have been shown to be an effective alternative for ventilating some newborns who have failed bag-and-mask ventilation or endotracheal intubation. However, there are limited data about the use of laryngeal mask airways (LMAs) for neonatal resuscitation. Experience with LMAs in preterm newborns and in meconium-stained newborns is even more limited. If your hospital uses LMAs, you will need to stock them on your resuscitation trays and personnel will require special training in their use. The details of LMA insertion will not be covered in this program.

What equipment and supplies are needed?

The supplies and equipment necessary to perform endotracheal intubation should be kept together and readily available. Each delivery room, nursery, and emergency department should have a complete set of the following items (Figure 5.1):

1. Laryngoscope with an extra set of batteries and extra bulbs.

2. Blades: No. 1 (term newborn), No. 0 (preterm newborn), No. 00 (optional for extremely preterm newborn). Straight rather than curved blades are preferred.

3. Endotracheal tubes with inside diameters of 2.5, 3.0, 3.5, and 4.0 mm.

4. Stylet (optional).

5. Carbon dioxide (CO_2) monitor or detector (optional).

6. Suction setup with 10F or larger suction catheter, plus sizes 5F or 6F and 8F for suctioning the endotracheal tube.

7. Roll of tape, 1/2 or 3/4 inch, or endotracheal tube securing device (optional).

8. Scissors.

9. Oral airway.

10. Meconium aspirator.

11. Stethoscope (neonatal head preferred).

12. Resuscitation bag and mask, manometer (optional), and oxygen tubing. Self-inflating bag must have oxygen reservoir.

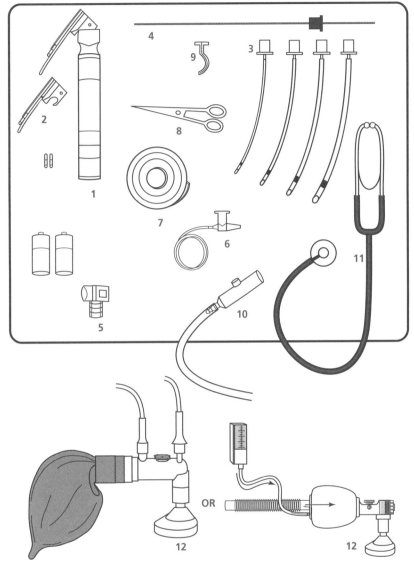

Figure 5.1. Neonatal resuscitation equipment and supplies

Intubation is best performed as a clean procedure. The endotracheal tubes and stylet should be clean and protected from contamination. The laryngoscope blades and handle should be thoroughly cleaned after each use.

What kind of endotracheal tubes are best to use?

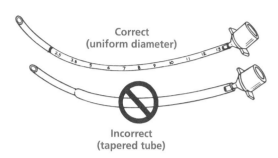

Figure 5.2. Endotracheal tubes with uniform diameter are preferred for newborns.

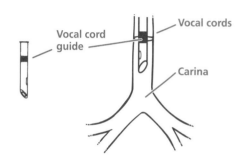

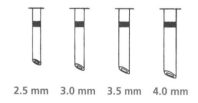

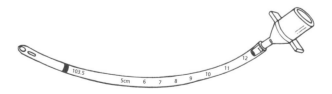

Figure 5.3. Characteristics of endotracheal tubes used for neonatal resuscitation

Sterile disposable tubes should be used. They should be of uniform diameter throughout the length of the tube, not tapered near the tip (Figure 5.2). One disadvantage of the tapered tube is that, during intubation, your view of the tracheal opening is easily obstructed by the wide part of the tube. Also, tubes with shoulders are more likely to become obstructed and cause trauma to the vocal cords.

Most endotracheal tubes for newborns have a black line near the tip of the tube, which is called a "vocal cord guide" (Figure 5.3). Such tubes are meant to be inserted so that the vocal cord guide is placed at the level of the vocal cords. This usually positions the tip of the tube above the bifurcation of the trachea (carina).

The length of the trachea in a premature newborn is less than that in a term newborn — 3 cm versus 5 to 6 cm. Therefore, the smaller the tube, the closer the vocal cord guide is to the tip of the tube.

Although tubes are available with cuffs at the level of the vocal cord guide, cuffs are not recommended when endotracheal intubation is required for resuscitation of newborns.

Endotracheal tubes made for newborns come with centimeter markings along the tube, identifying the distance from the tip of the tube. You will learn later to use these markings to identify the appropriate depth of insertion of the tube.

How do you prepare the endotracheal tube for use?

Select the appropriate-sized tube.

Tube Size (mm) (inside diameter)	Weight (g)	Gestational Age (wks)
2.5	Below 1,000	Below 28
3.0	1,000-2,000	28-34
3.5	2,000-3,000	34-38
3.5-4.0	Above 3,000	Above 38

Time will be limited once resuscitation is underway. Therefore, preparation of equipment *before* a high-risk delivery is important.

The approximate size of the endotracheal tube is determined from the baby's weight. The table gives the tube size for various weight and gestational age categories. Study the table. Later you will be asked to recall the suggested tube size for babies of various weights.

Consider cutting the tube to a shorter length.
Many endotracheal tubes come from the manufacturer much longer than necessary for orotracheal use. The extra length will increase resistance to airflow.

Some find it helpful to shorten the endotracheal tube before insertion (Figure 5.4). The endotracheal tube may be shortened to 13 to 15* cm to make it easier to handle during intubation and to lessen the chance of inserting the tube too far. A 13- to 15-cm tube will provide enough tube extending beyond the baby's lips for you to adjust the depth of insertion if necessary, and to properly secure the tube to the face. Remove the connector (note that the connection to the tube may be tight), and then cut the tube diagonally to make it easier to reinsert the connector.

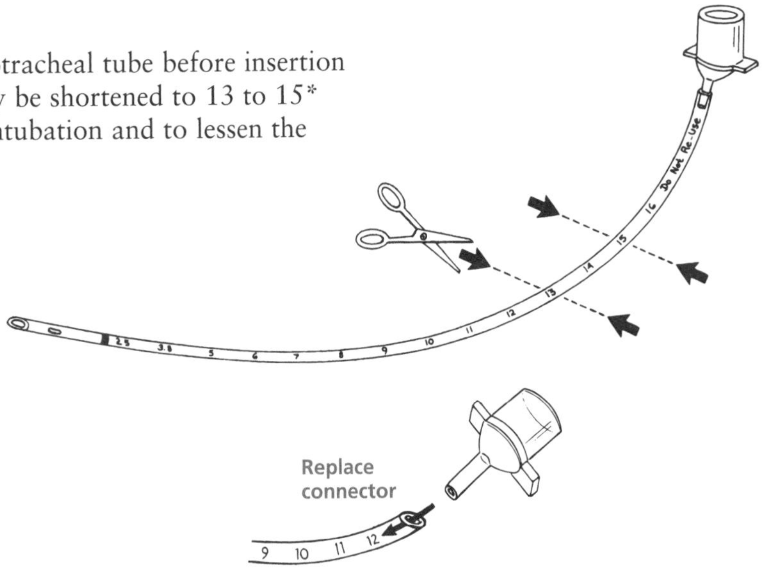

Replace connector

Replace the endotracheal tube connector. The fitting should be tight so that the connector does

Figure 5.4. Process of cutting endotracheal tube to length before insertion

not inadvertently separate during insertion or use. Connectors are made to fit a specific-sized tube. They cannot be interchanged between tubes of different sizes.

Others prefer to leave the tube long initially and then cut the tube to length after insertion if it is decided to leave it in place for longer than the immediate resuscitation.

*Note: The 15-cm length may be preferred to accommodate some types of endotracheal tube securing devices.

Use a stylet (optional).
Some people find it helpful to place a stylet through the endotracheal tube to provide rigidity and curvature to the tube, thus facilitating intubation (Figure 5.5). When inserting the stylet, it is essential that

- The tip does not protrude from the end or side hole of the endotracheal tube (to avoid trauma to the tissues).
- The stylet is secured so that it cannot advance farther into the tube during intubation.

Although many find the stylet helpful, others find the stiffness of the tube alone adequate. Use of a stylet is optional and depends on the operator's preference.

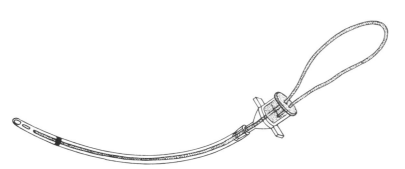

Figure 5.5. Optional stylet for increasing endotracheal tube stiffness and maintaining curvature during intubation

Caution: When stylets have been reused, they may have bends in them that make them fit very tightly in the endotracheal tube. Check to make certain that the stylet can be removed from the tube easily.

How do you prepare the laryngoscope and additional supplies?

Select blade and attach to handle.
First, select the appropriate-sized blade and attach it to the laryngoscope handle.

- No. 0 for preterm newborns
- No. 1 for term newborns

Check light.
Next, turn on the light to determine that the batteries and bulb are working. Check to see that the bulb is screwed in tightly to ensure that it will not flicker or fall out during the procedure.

Prepare suction equipment.
Suction equipment should be available and ready for use.

- Adjust the suction source to 100 mm Hg by occluding the end of the suction tubing.
- Connect a 10F (or larger) suction catheter to the suction tubing so that it will be available to suction secretions from the mouth and nose.
- Smaller suction catheters (5F, 6F, or 8F, depending on the size of the endotracheal tube) should be available for suctioning the tube if it becomes necessary to leave the endotracheal tube in place.

Endotracheal Tube Size	Catheter Size
2.5	5F or 6F
3.0	6F or 8F
3.5	8F
4.0	8F or 10F

Prepare resuscitation bag and mask.
A resuscitation bag and mask capable of providing 90% to 100% oxygen should be on hand to ventilate the baby between intubation attempts or if intubation is unsuccessful. The bag without the mask will be required to ventilate the baby after intubation to initially check tube placement and to provide continued ventilation if necessary. Check the operation of the bag as described in Lesson 3.

Turn on oxygen.
The oxygen tubing should be connected to an oxygen source and be available to deliver 100% free-flow oxygen and to connect to the resuscitation bag. The oxygen flow should be turned on to 5 to 10 L/min.

Get stethoscope.
A stethoscope will be needed to check for bilateral breath sounds.

Cut tape or prepare stabilizer.
Cut a strip of adhesive tape to secure the tube to the face, or prepare an endotracheal tube holder, if used at your hospital.

 Check yourself!

(The answers are in the preceding section and at the end of the lesson.)

1. A newborn with meconium and depressed respirations (will) (will not) require suctioning by endotracheal intubation before positive-pressure ventilation.

2. A newborn receiving ventilation by bag and mask is not improving after 2 minutes of apparently good technique. The chest is rising only slightly. Endotracheal intubation (should) (should not) be considered.

3. A newborn has not responded to ventilation and chest compressions and requires epinephrine to stimulate the heart. A common way to administer epinephrine directly into the trachea is through a(n) _____.

4. For babies weighing less than 1,000 g, the inside size of the endotracheal tube should be _____ mm.

5. The blade of a laryngoscope for preterm newborns should be No. _____. The blade for term newborns should be No. _____.

What anatomy do you need to know to insert the tube properly?

The anatomic landmarks that relate to intubation are labeled in Figures 5.6 through 5.8. Study the relative position of these landmarks, using all the figures, because each is important to your understanding of the procedure.

1. **Epiglottis** — A lidlike structure overhanging the entrance to the trachea
2. **Vallecula** — A pouch formed by the base of the tongue and the epiglottis
3. **Esophagus** — The food passageway extending from the throat to the stomach
4. **Cricoid** — Cartilage of the larynx
5. **Glottis** — The opening to the trachea; contains the vocal cords
6. **Vocal cords** — Folds of mucous membrane on both sides of the trachea, just within the glottis
7. **Trachea** — The windpipe or air passageway, extending from the throat to the main bronchi
8. **Main bronchi** — The two air passageways leading from the trachea to the lungs
9. **Carina** — Where the trachea branches into the two main bronchi

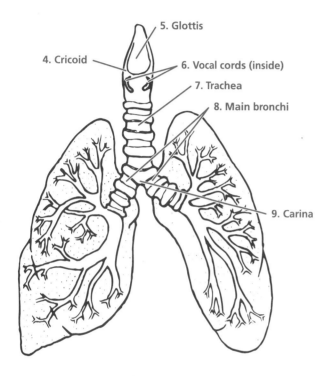

Figure 5.6. Anatomy of the airway

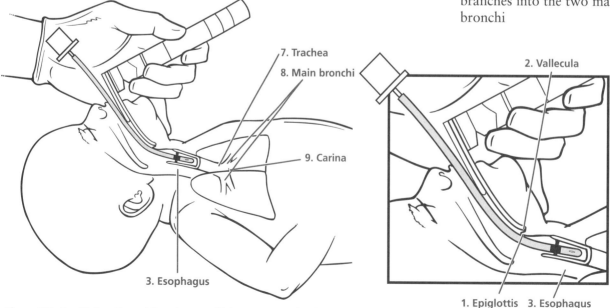

Figure 5.7. Sagittal section of the airway, with laryngoscope in place

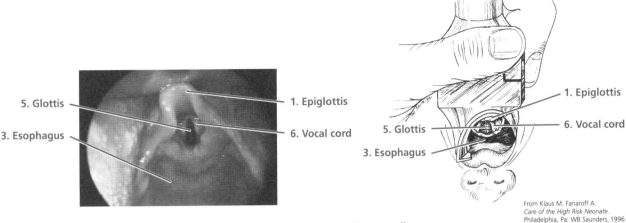

| 5. Glottis | | 1. Epiglottis |
| 3. Esophagus | | 6. Vocal cord |

	1. Epiglottis
5. Glottis	6. Vocal cord
3. Esophagus	

From Klaus M. Fanaroff A.
Care of the High Risk Neonate.
Philadelphia, Pa: WB Saunders, 1996

Figure 5.8. Photograph and drawing of laryngoscopic view of glottis and surrounding structures

How should you position the newborn to make intubation easiest?

The correct position of the newborn for intubation is the same as for bag-and-mask ventilation — on a flat surface with the head in a midline position and the neck slightly extended. It may be helpful to place a roll under the baby's shoulders to maintain slight extension of the neck.

This "sniffing" position aligns the trachea for optimal viewing by allowing a straight line of sight into the glottis once the laryngoscope has been properly placed (Figure 5.9).

It is important not to hyperextend the neck, because this will raise the glottis above your line of sight and narrow the trachea.

If there is too much flexion of the head toward the chest, you will be viewing the posterior pharynx and may not be able to directly visualize the glottis.

Correct — Line of sight clear (tongue will be lifted by laryngoscope blade)

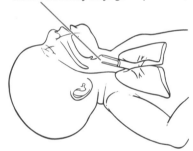

Incorrect — Line of sight obstructed

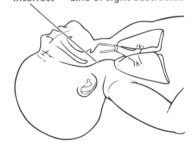

Incorrect — Line of sight obstructed

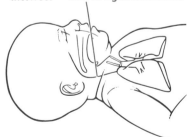

Figure 5.9. Correct (top) and incorrect (middle and bottom) positioning for intubation

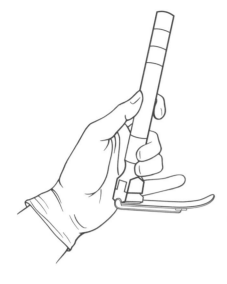

How do you hold the laryngoscope?

Turn on the laryngoscope light and hold the laryngoscope in your *left* hand, between your thumb and first two or three fingers, with the blade pointing away from you (Figure 5.10). One or two fingers should be left free to rest on the baby's face to provide stability.

The laryngoscope is designed to be held in the *left* hand — by both right- and left-handed persons. If held in the right hand, the closed curved part of the blade will block your view of the glottis, as well as make insertion of the endotracheal tube impossible.

Figure 5.10. Correct hand position when holding a laryngoscope for neonatal intubation

How do you visualize the glottis and insert the tube?

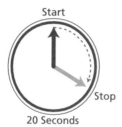

The next few steps will be described in detail. However, during an actual resuscitation, they will need to be completed very quickly — within approximately 20 seconds. The baby will not be ventilated during this process, so quick action is essential. Color photos of this procedure can be found on page C in the center section of the book.

First, stabilize the baby's head with your right hand (Figure 5.11). It may be helpful to have a second person hold the head in the desired "sniffing" position. Free-flow oxygen should be delivered throughout the procedure.

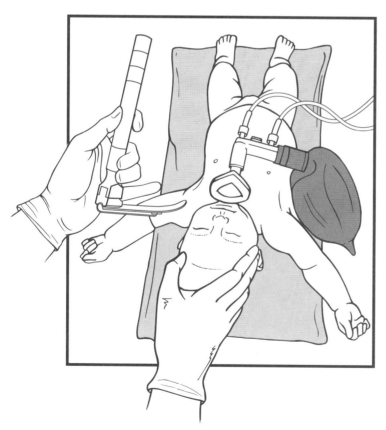

Figure 5.11. Preparing to insert the larynogoscope

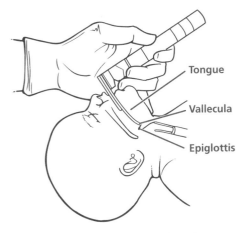

Figure 5.12. Landmarks for placement of the laryngoscope

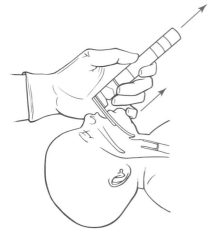

Figure 5.13. Lifting the laryngoscope blade to expose the opening of the larynx

Second, slide the laryngoscope blade over the right side of the tongue, pushing the tongue to the left side of the mouth, and advance the blade until the tip lies in the vallecula, just beyond the base of the tongue (Figure 5.12). You may need to use your right index finger to open the baby's mouth to make it easier to insert the laryngoscope.

Note: Although this lesson describes placing the tip of the blade in the vallecula, some prefer to place it directly on the epiglottis, gently compressing the epiglottis against the base of the tongue.

Third, lift the blade slightly, thus lifting the tongue out of the way to expose the pharyngeal area (Figure 5.13).

When lifting the blade, raise the *entire* blade by pulling up in the direction the handle is pointing (Figure 5.14).

 Do not elevate the tip of the blade by using a rocking motion and pulling the handle toward you.

Rocking rather than elevating the tip of the blade will not produce the view of the glottis you desire and will put excessive pressure on the alveolar ridge and possibly harm future tooth formation.

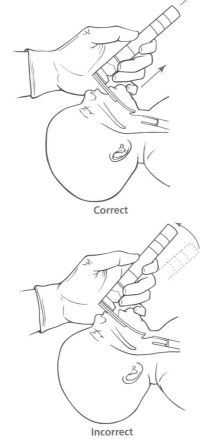

Correct

Incorrect

Figure 5.14. Correct (top) and incorrect (bottom) method for lifting the laryngoscope blade to expose the larynx

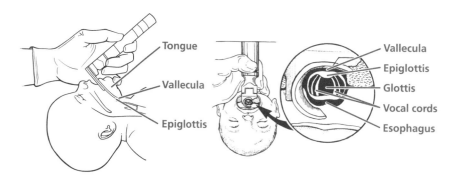

Figure 5.15. Identification of landmarks before placing endotracheal tube through glottis

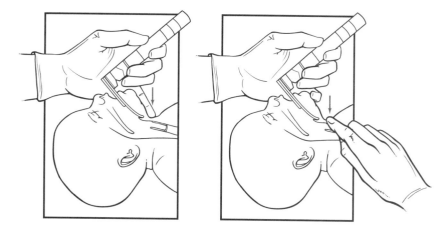

Figure 5.16. Improving visualization with pressure applied to larynx by intubator (left) or by an assistant (right)

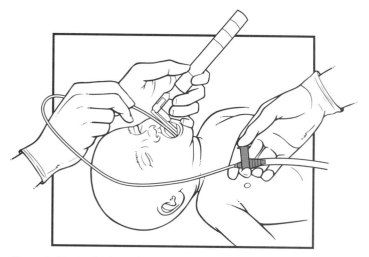

Figure 5.17. Suctioning of secretions

Fourth, look for landmarks (Figure 5.15). (Also, see color Figures C-2a, C-2b, C-2c, and C2d in the center of the book.)

If the tip of the blade is correctly positioned in the vallecula, you should see the epiglottis at the top, with the glottic opening below. You also should see the vocal cords appearing as vertical stripes on each side of the glottis or as an inverted letter "V" (Figure 5.8).

If these structures are not immediately visible, you should quickly adjust the blade until the structures come into view. Applying downward pressure to the cricoid (the cartilage that covers the larynx) may help bring the glottis into view (Figure 5.16). The pressure may be applied with your own little finger or by an assistant.

Suctioning of secretions also may be helpful to improve your view (Figure 5.17).

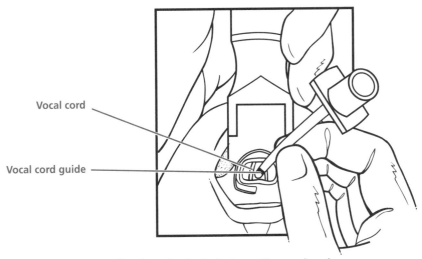

Figure 5.18. Insertion of endotracheal tube between the vocal cords

Fifth, insert the tube (Figure 5.18).

Holding the tube in your right hand, introduce it into the right side of the baby's mouth. This will prevent the tube from blocking your view of the glottis.

Keep the glottis in view and when the vocal cords are apart, insert the tip of the endotracheal tube until the vocal cord guide is at the level of the cords.

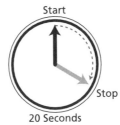

If the cords are together, wait for them to open. Do not touch the closed cords with the tip of the tube because it may cause spasm of the cords. If the cords do not open within 20 seconds, stop and ventilate with a bag and mask. After the heart rate and color have improved, you can then try again.

Be careful to insert the tube only so far as to place the vocal cord guide at the level of the vocal cords (Figure 5.19). This will position the tube in the trachea approximately halfway between the vocal cords and the carina.

Note the markings on the tube that align with the baby's lip.

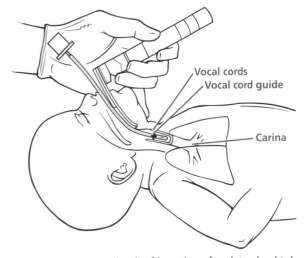

Figure 5.19. Correct depth of insertion of endotracheal tube

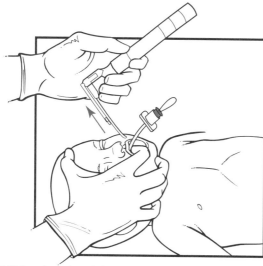

Figure 5.20. Stabilizing the tube while laryngoscope is withdrawn

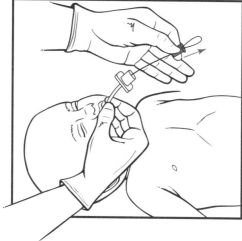

Figure 5.21. Removing stylet from endotracheal tube

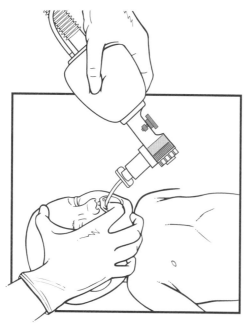

Figure 5.22. Resuming positive-pressure ventilation after endotracheal intubation

Sixth, stabilize the tube with one hand, and remove the laryngoscope with the other (Figure 5.20).

With the right hand held against the face, hold the tube *firmly* at the lips and/or use a finger to hold the tube against the baby's hard palate. Use your left hand to *carefully* remove the laryngoscope without displacing the tube.

If a stylet was used, remove it from the endotracheal tube — again be careful to hold the tube in place while you do so (Figure 5.21).

Although it is important to hold the tube firmly, be careful not to press the tube so tightly that the tube becomes compressed and obstructs airflow.

You are now ready to use the tube for the reason you inserted it.

• If the purpose was to **suction meconium,** then you should use the tube to suction meconium, as described on the next page.

• If the purpose was to **ventilate the baby,** then you should quickly attach a ventilation bag to the tube, take steps to be certain the tube is in the trachea, and resume positive-pressure ventilation with 100% oxygen (Figure 5.22).

What do you do next if the tube was inserted to suction meconium?

As described in Lesson 2, if there is meconium in the amniotic fluid and the baby has depressed muscle tone, depressed respirations, or a heart rate less than 100 beats per minute (bpm), the trachea should be intubated and suctioned.

As soon as the endotracheal tube has been inserted and the stylet, if used, has been removed,

- Connect the endotracheal tube to a meconium aspirator, which has been connected to a suction source (Figure 5.23). Several alternative types of meconium aspirators are available commercially, some of which include the endotracheal tube as part of the device.

- Occlude the suction-control port on the aspirator to apply suction to the endotracheal tube, and gradually withdraw the tube as you continue suctioning any meconium that may be in the trachea.

- Repeat intubation and suction as necessary until little additional meconium is recovered or until the baby's heart rate indicates that positive-pressure ventilation is needed.

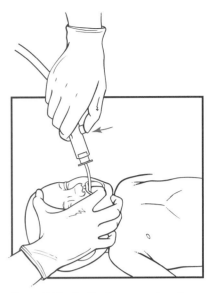

Figure 5.23. Suctioning meconium from trachea using an endotracheal tube, meconium aspiration device, and suction tubing connected to a suction source

For how long do you try to suction meconium?

Judgment is required when suctioning meconium. You have learned that you should suction the trachea only if the meconium-stained baby has depressed respirations or muscle tone or has a heart rate less than 100 bpm. Therefore, at the time you begin to suction the trachea, it is likely that the baby will already be significantly compromised and will eventually need resuscitation. You will need to delay resuscitation for a few seconds while you suction meconium, but you do not want to delay more than is absolutely necessary. The following are a few guidelines:

- Do not apply suction to the endotracheal tube for longer than 3 to 5 seconds as you withdraw the tube.

- If no meconium is recovered, don't repeat the procedure; proceed with resuscitation.

- If you recover meconium with the first suction, check the heart rate. If the baby does not have significant bradycardia, reintubate and suction again. If the heart rate is low, you may decide to administer positive pressure without repeating the procedure.

If you intubated to ventilate the baby, how do you check to be sure that the tube is in the trachea?

If the tube is positioned correctly, you should observe

• A rise in the chest with each breath

• Breath sounds over both lung fields but decreased or absent over the stomach (Figure 5.24)

• No gastric distention with ventilation

• Vapor condensing on the inside of the tube during exhalation

When listening to breath sounds, be sure to use a small stethoscope and place it laterally and high on the chest wall (in the axilla). Large stethoscopes, or a stethoscope placed too central or too low, may transmit sounds from the esophagus or stomach. Observe for a rise in the chest with each ventilated breath and for no gastric distension.

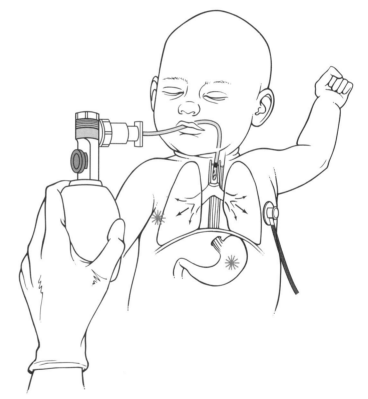

Figure 5.24. Breath sounds should be audible in both axillae but not over stomach. (See asterisks.)

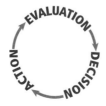

Be cautious when interpreting breath sounds in newborns. Since sounds are easily transmitted, those heard over the anterior portions of the chest may be coming from the stomach or esophagus. Breath sounds also can be transmitted to the abdomen.

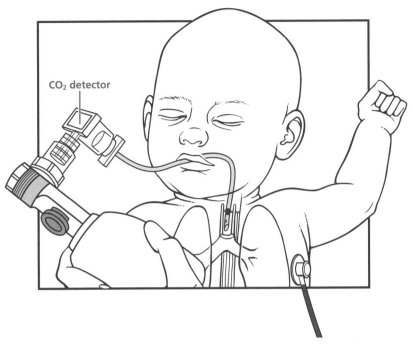

Figure 5.25. Carbon dioxide detector will change color during exhalation if endotracheal tube is in the trachea

Since the lungs are the primary organ for removal of CO_2 from the body, CO_2 levels will be much higher in the trachea than elsewhere in the body. Therefore, detection of the presence of CO_2 in the endotracheal tube can serve as confirmatory evidence that the tube is in the trachea rather than the esophagus (Figure 5.25). There are two basic types of CO_2 detectors available.

- Colorimetric devices are connected to the endotracheal tube and change color in the presence of CO_2.

- Capnographs rely on placement of a special electrode at the endotracheal tube connector. The capnograph will then display a specific CO_2 level and should read more than 2% to 3% CO_2 if the tube is in the trachea.

If you have any doubt about correct placement of the endotracheal tube, connect a CO_2 detector and note the presence or absence of CO_2 during exhalation. If CO_2 is not detected, consider removing the tube, resuming bag-and-mask ventilation, and repeating the intubation process as described on the next page.

 Caution: Extremely low-birthweight babies or babies with very poor cardiac output may exhale insufficient CO_2 to be detected reliably by CO_2 detectors.

What do you do if you suspect that the tube may *not* be in the trachea?

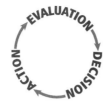

It is very important to be certain that the tube is in the trachea. A misplaced tube is worse than having no tube at all.

The tube is likely *not* in the trachea if you

- Do not see the chest rise.
- Do not hear good breath sounds over the lungs.
- Do hear air noises over the stomach.

or if

- There is no mist in the tube.
- The abdomen appears to become distended.
- The CO_2 monitor does not indicate the presence of exhaled CO_2.
- The newborn remains cyanotic and bradycardic despite positive-pressure ventilation.

If you suspect the tube is not in the trachea, you should do the following:

- Use your right hand to hold the tube in place while you use your left hand to reinsert the laryngoscope so that you can visualize the glottis and see if the tube is passing between the vocal cords.

and/or

- Remove the tube, use a bag and mask to stabilize the heart rate and color, and then repeat the intubation procedure.

Note: The CO_2 monitor may not change color if the cardiac output is very low or absent (eg, cardiac arrest). If there is no detectable heartbeat, do not use the CO_2 monitor as an indicator of correct or incorrect placement of the endotracheal tube.

How do you know if the tip of the tube is in the right location within the trachea?

If the tube is correctly placed, the tip will be located in the midtrachea, midway between the vocal cords and the carina (Figure 5.26). If it is in too far, it generally will be down the right main bronchus, and you will be ventilating only the right lung (Figure 5.27).

If the tube is correctly placed and the lungs are inflating, you will hear breath sounds of equal intensity on each side.

If the tube is in too far, you will hear breath sounds on the right side that are louder than any sounds you hear on the left side. If that is the case, pull back the tube very slowly while listening to the left side of the chest. When the tip reaches the carina, you should hear the breath sounds on the left increase.

You also can use the tip-to-lip measurement to estimate if the tube has been inserted the correct distance (see table). Adding 6 to the baby's weight in kilograms will give you a rough estimate of the correct distance from the tube tip to the vermillion border of the upper lip.

Weight (kg)	Depth of insertion (cm from upper lip)
1*	7
2	8
3	9
4	10

*Babies weighing less than 750 g may require only 6 cm insertion.

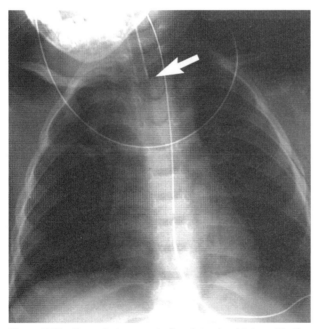

Figure 5.26. *Correct* placement of endotracheal tube with tip in midtrachea

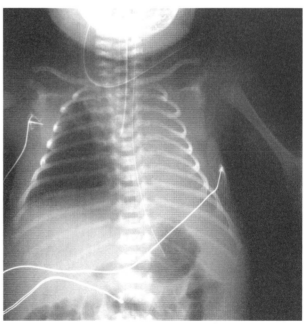

Figure 5.27. *Incorrect* placement of endotracheal tube with tip in right main bronchus. Note collapse of left lung.

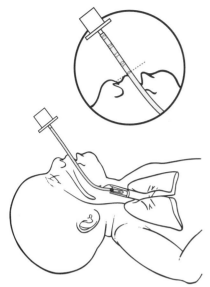

Figure 5.28. Measurement of endotracheal tube marking at the lip

After you have ensured that the tube is in the correct position, take note of the centimeter marking that appears at the upper lip. This can help you maintain the appropriate depth of insertion (Figure 5.28).

If you did not previously shorten the tube, it would be appropriate to do so now. However, be prepared to reinsert the connector quickly, as you will be unable to attach the resuscitation bag until you do so.

If the tube is going to be left in place beyond the initial resuscitation, you should obtain a chest x-ray as a final confirmation that the tube is in the proper position.

For long-term positive-pressure ventilation, the tube also will need to be secured to the face. However, description of this technique is beyond the scope of this program.

How do you continue resuscitation while you intubate?

Unfortunately, you will not be able to continue most resuscitation actions while you are intubating.

- Ventilation must be discontinued because the bag and mask must be removed from the airway during the procedure.
- Chest compressions generally must be interrupted because the movement of the baby created by the compressions will prevent you from seeing landmarks.

Therefore, you should make every effort to minimize the amount of hypoxia imposed during intubation. The following will be helpful:

- *Pre-oxygenate before attempting intubation.*
  Oxygenate the baby appropriately with bag and mask before beginning intubation and between repeated intubation attempts. This will not be possible when intubation is being performed for suctioning meconium or when a baby is being intubated to improve ventilation that was not effective with bag and mask.

- *Deliver free-flow oxygen during intubation.*
  Hold 100% free-flow oxygen by the baby's face while the intubator is clearing the airway and trying to visualize the landmarks. Then if the baby makes any spontaneous respiratory efforts during the procedure, he will be breathing oxygen-enriched air.

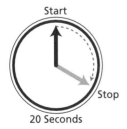

Start

Stop

20 Seconds

- *Limit attempts to 20 seconds.*
  Don't try to intubate for longer than approximately 20 seconds. If you are unable to visualize the glottis and insert the tube within 20 seconds, remove the laryngoscope and attempt to oxygenate the baby with bag-and-mask ventilation using 100% oxygen. Then try again.

What can go wrong while you are trying to intubate?

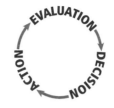

You may have trouble visualizing the glottis.

Problem	Landmarks	Corrective Action

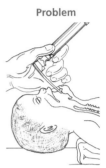 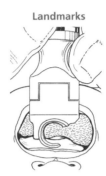 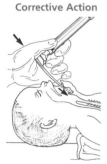

Laryngoscope not inserted far enough.

You see the tongue surrounding the blade.

Advance the blade farther.

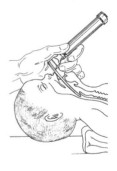 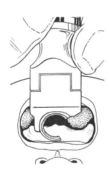 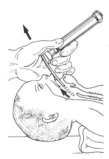

Laryngoscope inserted too far.

You see the walls of the esophagus surrounding the blade.

Withdraw the blade slowly until the epiglottis and glottis are seen.

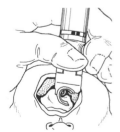 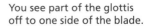 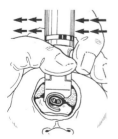

Laryngoscope inserted off to one side.

You see part of the glottis off to one side of the blade.

Gently move the blade back to the midline. Then advance or retreat according to landmarks seen.

Figure 5.29. Common problems associated with intubation

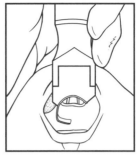
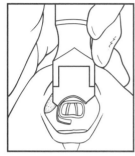

Figure 5.30. Poor visualization of the glottis (left) can be improved by elevating the tongue or depressing the larynx (right)

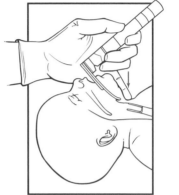
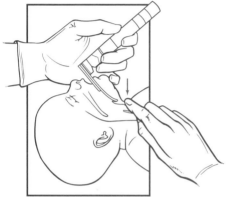

Figure 5.31. Improving visualization with pressure applied to larynx by intubator (left) or by an assistant (right)

Poor visualization of the glottis also may be caused by not elevating the tongue high enough to bring the glottis into view (Figure 5.30).

Sometimes, pressure applied to the cricoid, which is the cartilage covering the larynx, will help to bring the glottis into view (Figure 5.31).

This is accomplished by using the fourth or fifth finger of the left hand or by asking an assistant to apply the pressure.

You should practice intubating a manikin enough times so that you can find the correct landmarks quickly, thus allowing you to insert the tube within 20 seconds.

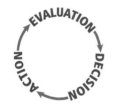

You may insert the tube into the esophagus instead of the trachea.

Having an endotracheal tube in the esophagus will be worse than having no tube at all, since the tube will tend to obstruct the baby's pharyngeal airway without providing an artificial airway. Therefore,

• Be certain that you visualize the glottis before inserting the tube. Watch the tube enter the glottis between the vocal cords.

• Look carefully for signs of esophageal intubation after the tube has been inserted. Use of a CO_2 detector can be very helpful.

If you have concerns that the tube may be in the esophagus, visualize the glottis and tube with a laryngoscope and/or remove the tube, oxygenate the newborn with a bag and mask, and reintroduce the tube.

> **Signs of endotracheal tube in esophagus**
>
> - Poor chest movement.
> - No breath sounds heard.
> - Air heard entering the stomach.
> - Gastric distention may be seen.
> - No mist in tube.
> - CO_2 detector fails to show presence of expired CO_2.
> - Poor response to intubation (cyanosis, bradycardia, etc).

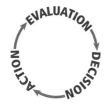

You may insert the tube too far into the trachea, down the right main bronchus.

If the tube is inserted too far, it usually will pass into the right main bronchus (Figure 5.32).

When you insert the tube, it is important to remember to watch the vocal cord guide on the tube and to stop inserting as soon as the guide reaches the cords.

Signs of the tube being in the right main bronchus include

- Breath sounds heard over the right but not the left side of the chest
- Louder breath sounds on the right side of the chest than on the left side
- Lack of improvement in the baby's color or heart rate

If you think the tube may be down the right main bronchus, first check the tip-to-lip measurement to see if the number at the lip may be higher than the estimated measurement from the table on page 5-19. Then withdraw the tube slightly while you listen over the left chest to hear if the breath sounds improve.

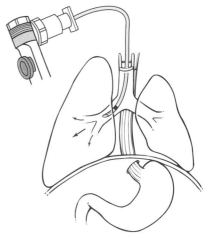

Figure 5.32. Endotracheal tube inserted too far (tip is down the right main bronchus)

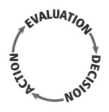

You may encounter other complications.

Complication	Possible Causes	Prevention or Corrective Action to Be Considered
Hypoxia	Taking too long to intubate	Pre-oxygenate with bag and mask. Provide free-flow oxygen during procedure. Halt intubation attempt after 20 seconds.
	Incorrect placement of tube	Reposition tube.
Bradycardia/apnea	Hypoxia Vagal response from laryngoscope or suction catheter	Pre-oxygenate with bag and mask. Provide free-flow oxygen during procedure. Oxygenate after intubation with bag and tube.
Pneumothorax	Overventilation of one lung due to tube in right main bronchus	Place tube correctly.
	Excessive ventilation pressures	Use appropriate ventilating pressures.
Contusions or lacerations of tongue, gums, or airway	Rough handling of laryngoscope or tube Inappropriate "rocking" rather than lifting of laryngoscope Laryngoscope blade too long or too short	Obtain additional practice/skill Select appropriate equipment.
Perforation of trachea or esophagus	Too vigorous insertion of tube Stylet protrudes beyond end of tube	Handle gently. Place stylet properly.
Obstructed endotracheal tube	Kink in tube or tube obstructed with secretions	Try to suction tube with catheter. If unsuccessful, consider replacing tube.
Infection	Introduction of organisms via hands or equipment	Pay careful attention to clean/sterile technique.

Lesson 5 Review

(The answers are at the end of the lesson.)

1. A newborn with meconium and depressed respirations (will) (will not) require suctioning by endotracheal intubation before positive-pressure ventilation.

2. A newborn receiving ventilation by bag and mask is not improving after 2 minutes of apparently good technique. The chest is rising only slightly. Endotracheal intubation (should) (should not) be considered.

3. A newborn has not responded to ventilation and chest compressions and requires epinephrine to stimulate the heart. A common way to administer epinephrine directly into the trachea is through a(n) _____.

4. For babies weighing less than 1,000 g, the inside size of the endotracheal tube should be _____ mm.

5. The blade of a laryngoscope for preterm newborns should be No. _____. The blade for term newborns should be No. _____.

6. Which illustration shows the view of the oral cavity that you should see if you have the laryngoscope correctly placed for intubation?

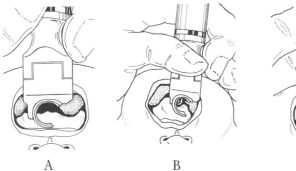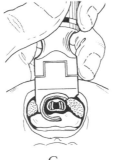

    A   B   C

Lesson 5 Review — *continued*

(The answers are at the end of the lesson.)

7. Both right- and left-handed people should hold the laryngoscope in their _____ hand.

8. You should take no longer than _____ seconds to complete endotracheal intubation.

9. If you have not completed endotracheal intubation within the time limit in Question 8, what should you do?

   _____

10. Which illustration shows the correct way to lift the tongue out of the way to expose the pharyngeal area?

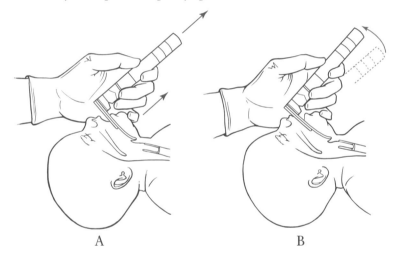

A   B

11. You have the glottis in view, but the vocal cords are closed. You (should) (should not) wait until they are open to insert the tube.

12. How far should the endotracheal tube be inserted into the baby's trachea?

   _____

Lesson 5 Review — *continued*

(The answers are at the end of the lesson.)

13. You have inserted an endotracheal tube and are giving positive-pressure ventilation through it. When you check with a stethoscope, you hear breath sounds on both sides of the baby's chest, with equal intensity on each side and no air entering the stomach. The tube (is) (is not) correctly placed.

14. Which x-ray shows the correct placement of an endotracheal tube?

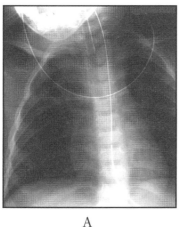
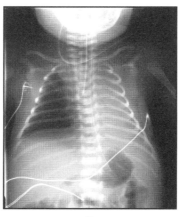

A   B

15. You have inserted an endotracheal tube and are giving positive-pressure ventilation through it. When you check with a stethoscope, you hear no breath sounds over either side of the chest and you hear air entering the stomach. The tube is placed in the (esophagus) (trachea).

16. If the tube is in the esophagus, it must be removed, the newborn given _____ by bag and mask, and the tube reinserted correctly.

17. You have inserted an endotracheal tube and are giving positive-pressure ventilation through it. When you check with a stethoscope, you hear breath sounds over the right side of the chest, but not the left. When you check the tip-to-lip measurement, it is higher than expected. You should (withdraw) (insert) the tube slightly and listen with the stethoscope again.

Performance Checklist
Lesson 5 — Endotracheal Intubation

Instructor: The learner should be instructed to talk through the procedure as it is demonstrated. Judge the performance of each step and check (✓) the box when the action is completed correctly. If done incorrectly, circle the box so that you can discuss that step later. You will need to provide information at several points concerning the condition of the baby.

Learner: To successfully complete this checklist, you should be able to perform all the steps and make all the correct decisions in the procedure. You should talk through the procedure as you perform it.

Equipment and Supplies

Intubation manikin

Radiant warmer or tabletop to simulate warmer

Gloves (or may be implied)

Stethoscope

Shoulder roll

Laryngoscope with fresh batteries and functioning light source

Blade, No. 1 (term) for use with manikin or No. 0 if appropriate

Endotracheal tubes, 2.5, 3.0, 3.5, 4.0 mm

Stylet (optional)

Tape or endotracheal tube securing device

Scissors (optional)

Mechanical suction device (or may be implied) with 10F or larger suction catheter

Self-inflating bag
   or
Flow-inflating bag with pressure manometer and oxygen source

Method to administer free-flow oxygen (oxygen mask, oxygen tubing, or flow-inflating bag and mask)

Flowmeter (or may simulate this)

Masks (term and preterm sizes)

Meconium aspirator

CO_2 detector (optional)

Clock with second hand

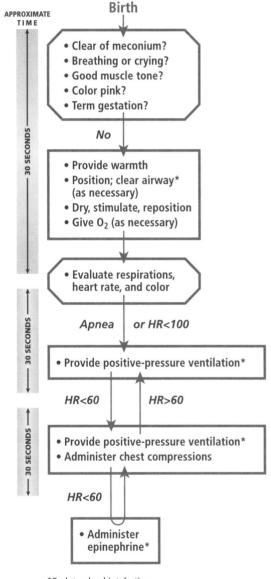

*Endotracheal intubation may be considered at several steps.

Performance Checklist
Lesson 5 — Endotracheal Intubation

Name _____ Instructor _____ Date _____

This performance checklist can be completed by learners who will be responsible for intubating and/or by those who will be assisting with intubation. If only one learner is being evaluated, the instructor may take the role of the other person.

Instructor's questions are in quotes. Learner's questions and correct responses are in bold type. Instructor should check boxes as the learner answers correctly.

Section A — Preparing for Intubation

"A full-term baby is about to be born. There have been severe fetal heart rate decelerations and there is meconium in the amniotic fluid. How would you prepare for this situation and assist with the activity?"

Endotracheal Tube

- [ ] **Selects correct-sized tube**
- [ ] **Cuts tube at 13 or 15 cm and replaces connector, securing a tight fit (optional)**
- [ ] **Inserts stylet (optional)**
  - [ ] **Stylet tip is *within* tip of tube**
  - [ ] **Secures stylet**

Laryngoscope

- [ ] **Selects appropriate-sized blade**
- [ ] **Attaches blade to laryngoscope and checks light — replaces batteries or bulb if necessary**

Additional Equipment

- [ ] **Obtains**
  - **• Oxygen tubing and source**
  - **• Suction equipment**
- [ ] **Obtains bag and mask**
  - [ ] **Checks bag for function**
  - [ ] **Prepares bag to give 90% to 100% oxygen**
  - [ ] **Selects appropriate-sized mask**
- [ ] **Obtains meconium aspiration device**
- [ ] **Cuts strip(s) of tape or prepares endotracheal tube securing device**

Section B — Performing or Assisting With Endotracheal Intubation

If you will be intubating rather than assisting, you will be asked to go through this procedure twice. The first time you should "talk through" the procedure, describing each action or observation made. This is necessary because your instructor is unable to view all aspects of the procedure directly.

The second time through, you will not need to describe what you are doing. Instead, work as quickly and efficiently as possible to complete the procedure within 20 seconds — from laryngoscope placement through tube insertion.

"The baby has just been born. Meconium was suctioned from the pharynx by the obstetrician before delivery of the shoulders, and the baby's skin is covered with meconium. She is placed under a radiant warmer and is limp. Demonstrate what you would do."

Performs Intubation   ## Assists

- [ ] Correctly positions manikin   [ ]
- [ ] Uses/provides free-flow oxygen   [ ]
- [ ] Provides suction when requested   [ ]
- [ ] Inserts blade into mouth, holding laryngoscope correctly
- [ ] Inserts blade just beyond tongue and lifts using correct motion
- [ ] Applies laryngeal pressure correctly when asked   [ ]
- [ ] Identifies landmarks seen
- [ ] Based on landmarks seen, takes corrective action if applicable
- [ ] Obtains unobstructed view of glottis
- [ ] Inserts tube into trachea
- [ ] Removes laryngoscope (and stylet if used) while firmly holding tube in place
- [ ] Connects (or assists with) meconium aspirator   [ ]
- [ ] Withdraws tube while applying suction
- [ ] Performs entire procedure within 20 seconds

"Assume that no further meconium is recovered during suctioning. The baby is limp and fails to resume spontaneous respirations following stimulation and several minutes of bag-and-mask ventilation. Although the baby is pink and has a heart rate greater than 100 bpm, you have decided to reinsert the endotracheal tube for continued positive-pressure ventilation."

Performs Intubation   Assists

☐ Administers positive-pressure ventilation with bag and mask   ☐

☐ Correctly positions manikin   ☐

☐ Uses/provides free-flow oxygen   ☐

☐ Provides suction when requested   ☐

☐ Inserts blade into mouth, holding laryngoscope correctly

☐ Inserts blade just beyond tongue and lifts using correct motion

☐ Applies laryngeal pressure correctly when asked   ☐

☐ Identifies landmarks seen

☐ Based on landmarks seen, takes corrective action if applicable

☐ Obtains unobstructed view of glottis

☐ Inserts tube, aligning vocal cord guide with vocal cords

☐ Removes laryngoscope (and stylet if used) while firmly holding tube so that tube position does not change

☐ Removes mask from bag and attaches to endotracheal tube and inflates lungs   ☐

☐ Consumes/notes no more than 20 seconds from blade insertion through correct tube placement   ☐

Provides Initial Confirmation of Placement

☐ Correctly states steps for confirming placement   ☐

☐ Observes chest rise with each breath

☐ Auscultates equal breath sounds over both lung fields but not over stomach

☐ Does not observe increasing gastric distension

☐ Observes vapor condensing on inside of tube during exhalation

☐ Considers use of CO_2 detector

"You have connected the resuscitation bag to the tube and resumed positive-pressure ventilation. However, the baby is cyanotic and the heart rate is 80 bpm."

☐ **Assesses need for corrective action and performs the necessary steps if tube is in esophagus or one of the bronchi**

   ☐ **Repeats confirmation steps**

   ☐ **Correctly assesses tip-to-lip measurement**

   ☐ **Reinserts laryngoscope and visualizes placement of stripe at vocal cords**

      and/or

   ☐ **Removes endotracheal tube, ventilates with bag and mask, and repeats intubation**

"The baby's color has improved and the heart rate is now greater than 100 bpm. However, the baby remains apneic and you have decided to leave the tube in place during transfer to ongoing care."

Takes Final Steps

   ☐ **States centimeter marking at level of upper lip**

   ☐ **Secures tube while maintaining proper position**
   (technique will depend on specific method used in learner's hospital)

   ☐ **Shortens tube if more than 4 cm extends from lips**

Overall Assessment

   ☐ **Gently handles baby, laryngoscope, and endotracheal tube to prevent trauma**

   ☐ **Limits attempts to 20 seconds**

Key Points

1. A person experienced in endotracheal intubation should be available to assist at every delivery.

2. Indications for endotracheal intubation include the following:

   - To suction trachea in presence of meconium when the newborn is not vigorous
   - To improve efficacy of ventilation after several minutes of bag-and-mask ventilation or ineffective bag-and-mask ventilation
   - To facilitate coordination of chest compressions and ventilation and to maximize the efficiency of each ventilation
   - To administer epinephrine if required to stimulate the heart

3. The laryngoscope is always held in the operator's left hand.

4. The correct-sized laryngoscope blade for a term newborn is No. 1. The correct-sized blade for a preterm newborn is No. 0.

5. The intubation procedure should be completed within 20 seconds.

6. The steps for intubating a newborn are as follows:

   - Stabilize the newborn's head in the "sniffing" position. Deliver free-flow oxygen during procedure.
   - Slide laryngoscope over the right side of the tongue, pushing the tongue to the left side of the mouth, and advancing the blade until the tip lies just beyond the base of the tongue.
   - Lift the blade slightly. Raise the entire blade, not just the tip.
   - Look for landmarks. Vocal cords should appear as vertical stripes on each side of the glottis or as an inverted letter "V".
   - Suction if necessary for visualization.
   - Insert the tube into the right side of the mouth.
   - If the cords are closed, wait for them to open. Insert the tip of the endotracheal tube until the vocal cord guide is at the level of the cords.
   - Hold the tube firmly against the baby's palate while removing the laryngoscope. Hold the tube in place while removing the stylet if one was used.

7. Correct placement of the endotracheal tube in the midtrachea is indicated by

   - A rise in the chest with each breath
   - Breath sounds over both lung fields but decreased or absent over the stomach
   - No gastric distention with ventilation
   - Vapor in the tube during exhalation
   - Presence of exhaled CO_2 as determined by a CO_2 detector
   - Tip-to-lip measurement: add 6 to newborn's weight in kilograms
   - Chest x-ray confirmation if tube is to remain in place past initial resuscitation
   - Direct visualization of the tube passing between the vocal cords

Answers to Questions

1. A newborn with meconium and depressed respirations **will** require suctioning by endotracheal intubation before positive-pressure ventilation.

2. Endotracheal intubation **should** be considered for a newborn who is not improving despite good technique.

3. A common way to administer epinephrine directly into the trachea is through an **endotracheal tube.**

4. For babies weighing less than 1,000 g, the inside size of the endotracheal tube should be **2.5** mm.

5. The blade of a laryngoscope should be No. **0** for preterm newborns and No. **1** for term newborns.

6. Illustration **C** shows the correct view for intubation.

7. Both right- and left-handed people should hold the laryngoscope in their **left** hand.

8. You should get an endotracheal tube inserted and connected to a bag in **20 seconds.**

9. If you have not completed endotracheal intubation within 20 seconds, you should **remove the laryngoscope, ventilate with bag and mask, and then try again.**

10. Illustration **A** is correct.

11. You **should** wait until the vocal cords are open to insert the tube.

12. You should insert the tube **to the level of the vocal cord guide.**

13. The tube **is** correctly placed.

14. X-ray **A** shows correct placement of an endotracheal tube.

15. The tube is placed in the **esophagus.**

16. The newborn should be given **ventilation** by bag and mask. The tube should then be reinserted correctly.

17. You should **withdraw** the tube slightly and listen with the stethoscope again.

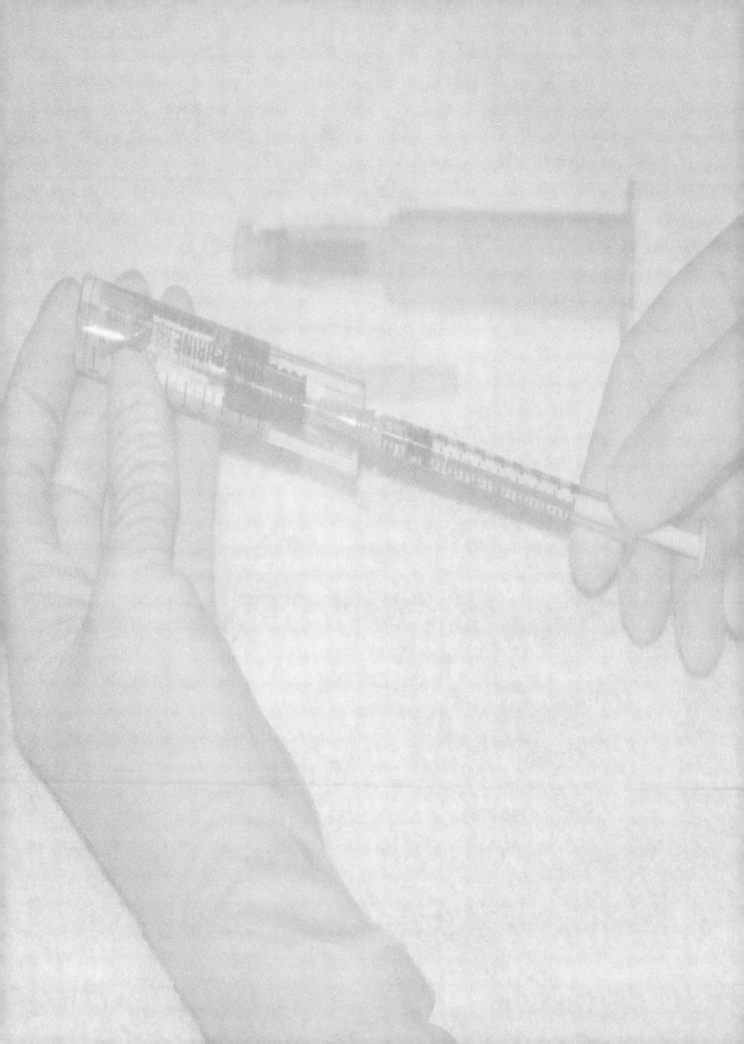

Medications

In Lesson 6 you will learn

• When to give medications during a resuscitation

• How to administer epinephrine through an
  – Endotracheal tube
  – Umbilical vein

• When and how to administer fluids intravenously to expand blood volume during a resuscitation

• When and how to administer sodium bicarbonate to correct metabolic acidosis during a resuscitation

The following case is an example of how medications may be used during an extensive resuscitation. As you read the case, imagine yourself as part of the resuscitation team. The details of this step will be described in the remainder of the lesson.

Case 5. Resuscitation with positive-pressure ventilation, chest compressions, and medications

A pregnant woman enters the emergency department complaining of the sudden onset of intense abdominal pain associated with contractions.

An ultrasound discloses a partial placental abruption, and persistent fetal bradycardia is noted. Additional skilled personnel are called to the delivery room, the radiant warmer is turned on, and resuscitation equipment is prepared. An emergency cesarean section is performed and a limp, pale baby is given to the neonatal team.

The team positions her head, suctions her mouth and nose, and stimulates her with drying. However, the baby remains limp, cyanotic, and without spontaneous respirations.

The team gives her positive-pressure ventilation with a bag and mask using 100% oxygen. However, after 30 seconds she remains cyanotic and limp and has a very low heart rate (20 to 30 beats per minute [bpm]).

The team begins chest compressions interposed with positive-pressure ventilation. Repeated assessments are made to be certain that the airway is clear, and the head is positioned so that ventilation is adequately moving the chest. Nevertheless, after another 30 seconds, the heart rate has not increased.

The team rapidly intubates the trachea to ensure effective ventilation, and epinephrine is instilled into the endotracheal tube. The heart rate is checked every 30 seconds as coordinated chest compressions and positive-pressure ventilation are continued.

After 3 minutes, another dose of epinephrine is given. Because the baby has persistent bradycardia and a history of possible blood loss, the umbilical vein is cannulated, and 30 mL of normal saline is given (weight is estimated at 3 kg). The heart rate gradually increases. By 7 minutes after birth, the baby makes an initial gasp. Chest compressions are stopped when the heart rate is noted to rise above 60 bpm. Assisted ventilation is continued with 100% oxygen and the heart rate rises above 100 bpm. The baby's color begins to improve, and she begins to show some spontaneous respirations.

She is transferred to the nursery for ongoing care.

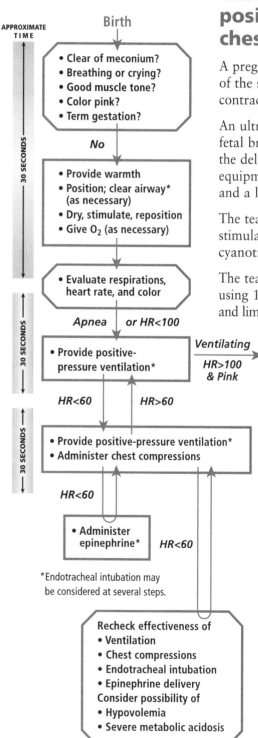

APPROXIMATE TIME

30 SECONDS

Birth

- Clear of meconium?
- Breathing or crying?
- Good muscle tone?
- Color pink?
- Term gestation?

No

- Provide warmth
- Position; clear airway* (as necessary)
- Dry, stimulate, reposition
- Give O₂ (as necessary)

- Evaluate respirations, heart rate, and color

Apnea or *HR<100*

30 SECONDS

- Provide positive-pressure ventilation*

Ventilating HR>100 & Pink → **Ongoing care**

HR<60 | *HR>60*

30 SECONDS

- Provide positive-pressure ventilation*
- Administer chest compressions

HR<60

- Administer epinephrine*

HR<60

*Endotracheal intubation may be considered at several steps.

Recheck effectiveness of
- Ventilation
- Chest compressions
- Endotracheal intubation
- Epinephrine delivery
Consider possibility of
- Hypovolemia
- Severe metabolic acidosis

If resuscitation steps have been implemented in a skillful and timely manner, more than 99% of newborns requiring resuscitation will have improved without the need for medications. By this point you should have checked the effectiveness of ventilation several times, ensuring that there is good chest rise with each breath. As part of this assessment, you may have inserted an endotracheal tube to be certain there is a good airway and so chest compressions and ventilation can more easily be coordinated.

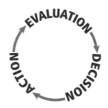 **If the heart rate remains below 60 bpm despite administration of ventilation and chest compressions, your first action should be to ensure that ventilation and compressions are being given optimally and that you are using 100% oxygen.**

However, despite good ventilation of the lungs with positive-pressure ventilation and improved cardiac output from chest compressions, a small number of newborns (fewer than 2 per 1,000 births) will still have a heart rate below 60 bpm. The heart muscle of these babies may have been deprived of oxygen for so long that it will not contract effectively despite now being perfused with oxygenated blood. These babies may benefit from receiving epinephrine to stimulate the heart. If there has been acute blood loss, they may benefit from volume replacement.

What will this lesson cover?

This lesson will teach you when to give *epinephrine*, how to establish a route by which to give it, and how to determine dosage.

The lesson also will discuss special medications that may be helpful to support the circulation.

- *Volume expansion* for babies in shock from blood loss
- *Sodium bicarbonate* for babies who have severe metabolic acidosis

Administration of naloxone, a narcotic antagonist given to babies who have depressed respirations from maternal narcotics, is not necessary during the acute phases of resuscitation and will be discussed in Lesson 7. Other drugs, such as atropine and calcium, are sometimes used during special resuscitation circumstances, but are not indicated in routine neonatal resuscitation. Studies have shown these and some other drugs to be of no value and perhaps damaging in the acute phase of neonatal resuscitation. Calcium may be useful in specific situations, such as hypocalcemia and hyperkalemia, but these situations are rare in the immediate newborn period and are not considerations during the acute phase of delivery room resuscitation.

When should epinephrine be given?

You have already learned that epinephrine is indicated when the heart rate remains below 60 bpm after you have given 30 seconds of assisted ventilation and another 30 seconds of coordinated chest compressions and ventilation.

Epinephrine is not indicated before you have established adequate ventilation because

- You will be wasting valuable time that should be focused on establishing effective ventilation and oxygenation.
- Epinephrine will increase workload and oxygen consumption of the heart muscle, which, in the absence of available oxygen, may cause unnecessary myocardial damage.

PREMATURITY POINTERS
Avoid using very high doses of epinephrine in the preterm baby. The potential hypertension and increased cerebral blood flow from residual epinephrine, after the heart rate improves, may be associated with bleeding in the fragile germinal matrix.

How should epinephrine be given?

Epinephrine should be given by the most accessible route that will deliver the drug to the heart muscle. The heart muscle receives blood from the coronary arteries, which are located just beyond the left ventricle. Therefore, epinephrine should be given into blood that will rapidly drain into the heart. In the newborn, the most accessible routes are

- **The endotracheal tube.** Epinephrine given into the endotracheal tube will be absorbed by the lungs into the pulmonary veins, which drain directly into the heart. Although this is generally the most accessible route, the requirement for absorption by the lungs makes the response time slower than if epinephrine is given directly into the blood.
- **The umbilical vein.** Epinephrine given into a catheter placed in the umbilical vein will enter the inferior vena cava, which drains into the right atrium of the heart. Although this route is likely associated with more effective blood levels of the drug, additional time is required to insert the catheter.

How do you give epinephrine through an endotracheal tube?

Epinephrine can be injected directly into the endotracheal tube (Figure 6.1, left). The medication is then forced into the lungs during positive-pressure ventilation.

One problem with this method of administration is that the small volume of drug injected into the relatively large endotracheal tube may collect in the connector, thus not reaching the lung for absorption. A small volume of normal saline (0.5 to 1.0 mL) may be used to flush the epinephrine down the tube.

To be sure the drug reaches the lungs, some providers prefer to inject the drug into a 5F feeding tube that has been inserted down the endotracheal tube (Figure 6.1, right). After injecting the medication, the feeding tube is then flushed with enough normal saline to clear the medication from the feeding tube (0.5 mL for a 15-inch 5F tube). The feeding tube is then removed and positive-pressure ventilation provided to distribute the medication into the bronchial tree.

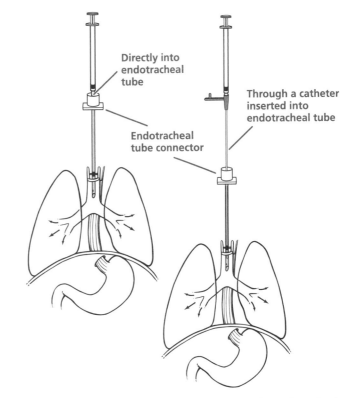

Figure 6.1. Epinephrine may be administered directly into the endotracheal tube (left) or through a catheter inserted into the endotracheal tube (right).

With either technique, rather than "chasing" the dose of epinephrine with saline, the desired dose of the medication can be diluted with normal saline to the full syringe volume (1 mL) before injection into the endotracheal tube or the catheter.

Note: Although an endotracheal tube is usually the most accessible route, medication absorption through the lungs during a neonatal resuscitation is not well studied and may lead to low plasma concentrations. If medications are needed in a resuscitation, efforts should be made to establish intravenous access (usually the umbilical vein), especially in a newborn who fails to respond to medications administered through an endotracheal tube.

 Caution: In Lesson 7 you will learn that another drug, naloxone, also may be given through an endotracheal tube. However, other drugs, such as sodium bicarbonate, are very caustic and, in large doses, will burn the sensitive lung tissue. These caustic drugs must be given slowly into a large blood vessel where they will be quickly diluted, NOT into an endotracheal tube.

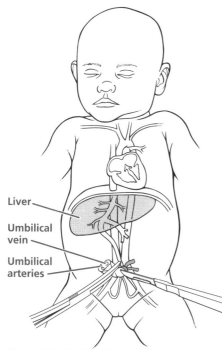

Liver

Umbilical vein

Umbilical arteries

Figure 6.2. Cutting the umbilical stump in preparation for inserting umbilical catheter

How do you give epinephrine through the umbilical vein?

The umbilical vein is readily accessible in the newborn.

- Place a loose tie of umbilical tape around the base of the cord. This tie can be tightened if there is excessive bleeding after you cut the cord. Clean the cord with povidone-iodine.

- Pre-fill a 3.5F or 5F umbilical catheter with normal saline. The catheter should have a single end-hole and be connected to a stopcock and syringe. Close the stopcock to the catheter to prevent fluid loss and air entry.

- Using sterile technique, cut the cord with a scalpel below the clamp and about 1 to 2 cm from the skin line (Figure 6.2). Make the cut perpendicular rather than at an angle. The umbilical vein will be seen as a large, thin-walled structure, usually at the 11- to 12-o'clock position. The two umbilical arteries have thicker walls and usually lie close together somewhere in the 4- to 8-o'clock position. However, the arteries coil within the cord. Therefore, the longer the cord stump below your cut, the greater the likelihood that the vessels will not lie in the positions described.

- Insert the catheter into the umbilical vein (Figure 6.3). The course of the vein will be up, toward the heart, so this is the direction you should point the catheter. Continue inserting the catheter 2 to 4 cm (less in preterm babies) until you get free flow of blood when you open the stopcock between the catheter and the syringe and the syringe is gently aspirated. For emergency use during resuscitation, the tip of the catheter should be located only a short distance into the vein — when blood is first able to be aspirated. If the catheter is inserted farther, there is risk of infusing solutions into the liver and possibly causing damage.

- Inject the appropriate dose of epinephrine (see next page), followed by 0.5- to 1.0-mL normal saline to clear the drug from the catheter into the baby.

- Once the baby has been fully resuscitated, either suture the catheter in place or remove the catheter, tighten the cord tie, and complete the knot to prevent bleeding from the umbilical stump. Do not advance the catheter once the sterile field has been violated.

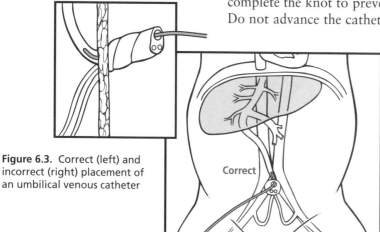
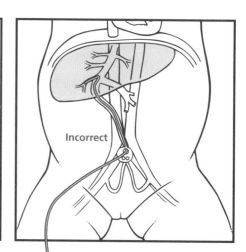

Correct

Incorrect

Figure 6.3. Correct (left) and incorrect (right) placement of an umbilical venous catheter

What is epinephrine, how should you prepare it, and how much should you give?

Epinephrine hydrochloride (sometimes referred to as adrenaline chloride) is a cardiac stimulant. Epinephrine increases the strength and rate of cardiac contractions and causes peripheral vasoconstriction, which may play a role in increasing blood flow through the coronary arteries and to the brain.

Although epinephrine is available in both 1:1,000 and 1:10,000 concentrations, the 1:10,000 concentration is recommended for newborns, eliminating the need to dilute the 1:1,000 concentration.

Recommended concentration = 1:10,000

The endotracheal route may result in lower blood concentrations by the time the drug reaches the heart. Intravenous epinephrine may be more effective, but delivery may be delayed by the time required to establish intravenous access.

Recommended route = by endotracheal tube or intravenously

The recommended dose in newborns is 0.1 to 0.3 mL/kg of a 1:10,000 solution (equal to 0.01 to 0.03 mg/kg). You will need to estimate the baby's weight after birth. The endotracheal route may be associated with lower blood levels of the drug. Therefore, you might consider using the higher end of the dosage range when using this route. Considerably higher doses have been suggested for adults and older children when they do not respond to a lower dose. However, there is no evidence that this results in a better outcome. There is some concern that higher doses in babies may result in brain and heart damage.

Recommended dose = 0.1 to 0.3 mL/kg of 1:10,000 solution

Recommended preparation = 1:10,000 solution in 1-mL syringe

When giving epinephrine by endotracheal tube, be sure to give the drug directly into the tube, being careful not to leave it deposited in the endotracheal tube connector or adhered to the walls of the tube. Some people prefer to use a catheter to give the drug deeply into the tube. Whether the drug is given through an endotracheal tube or a catheter, you may decide to flush the drug in with 0.5 to 1.0 mL of normal saline. You should follow the drug with several deep, positive-pressure breaths to distribute the drug throughout the lungs for absorption.

Recommended rate of administration = *Rapidly* — as quickly as possible

Check yourself!

(The answers are in the preceding section and at the end of the lesson.)

1. Most babies who need resuscitation will respond to positive-pressure ventilation and chest compressions. However, a small number will have heart rates below 60 beats per minute after 90 seconds of resuscitation. Fewer than _____ babies per 1,000 births will need epinephrine to stimulate their hearts.

2. Ninety seconds into a resuscitation, a baby's heart rate is less than 60 beats per minute. You should now give _____ by the most quickly accessible route while continuing chest compressions and _____.

3. Which drugs should NOT be administered through an endotracheal tube?
   ____Epinephrine   ____Naloxone   ____Sodium bicarbonate

4. A newborn is intubated and is receiving positive-pressure ventilation and chest compressions. If you want to administer epinephrine quickly, which route should you choose?
   ____Endotracheal tube   ____Umbilical vein

5. You may follow an injection of endotracheal epinephrine with an injection of _____ _____ to ensure that most of the drug is delivered to the baby and not left in the catheter or tube.

6. Epinephrine is a cardiac (stimulant) (depressant).

7. Epinephrine (increases) (decreases) the strength of cardiac contractions and (increases) (decreases) the rate of cardiac contractions.

8. The recommended concentration of epinephrine for newborns is (1:1,000) (1:10,000).

9. The recommended dose of epinephrine for newborns is ___ mL/kg of a 1:10,000 solution.

10. Epinephrine should be given (slowly) (as quickly as possible).

What should you expect to happen after giving epinephrine?

As you continue positive-pressure ventilation and chest compressions, the heart rate should increase to more than 60 bpm within 30 seconds after you give epinephrine.

If this does not happen, you can repeat the dose every 3 to 5 minutes. However, you also should ensure that

- There is good chest movement and there are bilateral breath sounds.

- Chest compressions are given to a depth of one third the diameter of the chest and are well coordinated with ventilations.

- An endotracheal tube is placed, if one has not already been inserted. If a tube has been placed, ensure that the tube has remained in the trachea during cardiopulmonary resuscitation activities.

- The epinephrine has reached the baby's heart. Consider that the drug may still be in the endotracheal tube. You may decide to insert an umbilical catheter to ensure vascular delivery, and you may decide to repeat the epinephrine dose.

If the baby is pale and there is evidence of blood loss, you also may consider the possibility of volume loss. By this point the baby also is likely to have developed metabolic acidosis. Treatment of hypovolemia and acidosis will be covered next.

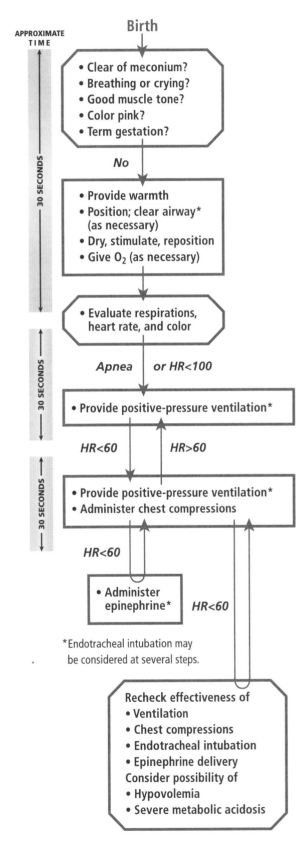

What should you do if the baby is pale, there is evidence of blood loss, and/or the baby is responding poorly to resuscitation?

If there has been a placental abruption, a placenta previa, or blood loss from the umbilical cord, the baby may be in hypovolemic shock. In some cases, the baby may have lost blood into the maternal circulation and there will be signs of shock with no obvious evidence of blood loss.

Babies in shock will appear pale and have weak pulses. They may have a persistently high or persistently low heart rate, and circulatory status often will not improve in response to effective ventilation, chest compressions, and epinephrine.

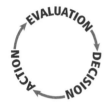

If the baby is not responding to resuscitation and there is evidence of blood loss, administration of a volume expander may be indicated.

What can you give to expand blood volume? How much should you give? How can you give it?

The recommended solution for acutely treating hypovolemia is an isotonic crystalloid solution. Acceptable solutions include

- Normal saline.
- Ringer's lactate.
- O-negative blood, cross-matched with mother's blood if time permits. (This sometimes may be prepared before the delivery if prenatal diagnosis has suggested low fetal blood volume.) If very large-volume blood loss is suspected, emergency-release O-negative blood may be necessary.

Recommended solution =
Normal saline

The initial dose is 10 mL/kg. However, if the baby shows minimal improvement after the first dose, you may need to give another dose of 10 mL/kg.

Recommended dose =
10 mL/kg

Volume expander must be given into the vascular system. The umbilical vein is usually the most accessible vein in a newborn, although the intraosseous route can be used.

Recommended route =
Umbilical vein

If hypovolemia is suspected, you should fill a large syringe with normal saline or other volume expander while others on the team continue resuscitation.

Recommended preparation =
Estimated volume drawn into large syringe

Although hypovolemia should be corrected fairly quickly, some clinicians are concerned that rapid administration in a newborn may result in intracranial hemorrhage.

Recommended rate of administration =
Over 5 to 10 minutes

PREMATURITY POINTERS
Preterm babies have a very fragile network of capillaries in the germinal matrix of their brains. Therefore, they are at particularly high risk of developing intracranial hemorrhage from too rapid administration of blood volume expanders.

What can you give if severe metabolic acidosis is suspected or has been proven from blood gas analysis?

Although the use of sodium bicarbonate during resuscitation is controversial, it may be helpful to correct metabolic acidosis that has resulted from a buildup of lactic acid. Lactic acid is formed when tissues have had insufficient oxygen. Severe acidosis will cause the myocardium to contract poorly and will cause the blood vessels of the lungs to constrict, thus decreasing pulmonary blood flow and preventing the lungs from adequately oxygenating the blood.

However, sodium bicarbonate can be harmful, particularly if given too early in a resuscitation. You should be certain that ventilation of the lungs is adequate. When sodium bicarbonate mixes with acid, carbon dioxide (CO_2) is formed. The lungs must be adequately ventilated to remove the CO_2.

Do not give sodium bicarbonate unless the lungs are being adequately ventilated.

Note: Although it is not unusual for metabolic acidosis to be found in a severely compromised baby, the condition will usually self-resolve with restoration of adequate circulating volume and adequate oxygenation. Some clinicians believe that bicarbonate therapy should be delayed until a blood gas analysis confirms a significant metabolic acidosis and a normal level of CO_2.

How much sodium bicarbonate should you give? How should you give it?

Recommended dose =
2 mEq/kg (4 mL/kg of 4.2% solution)

Recommended route =
Umbilical vein, from which there is good blood return

Recommended preparation =
0.5 mEq/mL (4.2% solution)

Recommended rate of administration =
Slowly — no faster than a rate of 1 mEq/kg/min

Sodium bicarbonate may be given if all other steps of resuscitation have been taken and there is still no improvement. If you decide to give sodium bicarbonate, remember that it is very caustic and hypertonic and, therefore, must be given into a large vein, from which there is good blood return.

Sodium bicarbonate is very caustic and should NOT be given through the endotracheal tube during resuscitation.

Sodium bicarbonate (4.2%) is commercially available in prefilled 10-mL syringes.

Sodium bicarbonate corrects metabolic acidosis by producing CO_2 and water. There must be adequate time for ventilation to remove the CO_2 produced. Because of this and the hypertonicity, the drug should be given slowly — no faster than 1 mEq/kg/min.

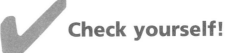

Check yourself!

(The answers are in the preceding section and at the end of the lesson.)

11. What should you do approximately 30 seconds after giving epinephrine?

12. If the baby's heart rate remains below 60 beats per minute, you can repeat the dose of epinephrine every _____ to _____ minutes.

13. If the baby's heart rate remains below 60 beats per minute after you have given epinephrine, you also should check to make sure that ventilation is producing good chest movement and that _____ _____ are being done correctly.

14. If the baby is pale, there is evidence of blood loss, and resuscitation is not resulting in improvement, you should consider giving _____ mL/kg of _____ by _____ .

15. Two characteristics of sodium bicarbonate are hypertonicity and conversion to CO_2. These factors encourage what precautions when giving it during resuscitation?
    (1) _____
    (2) _____
    (3) _____

16. Which route of delivery is contraindicated for giving sodium bicarbonate during resuscitation?_____ .

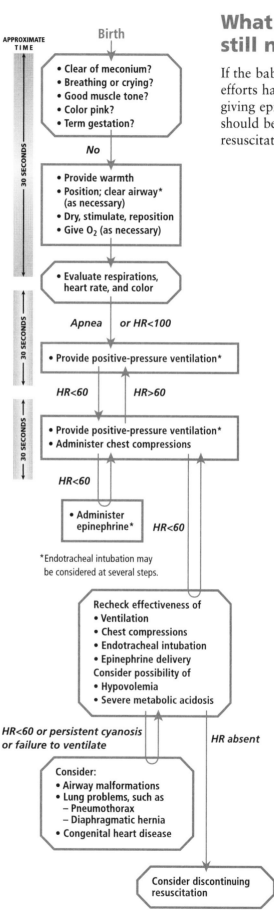

APPROXIMATE TIME

Birth

30 SECONDS

- Clear of meconium?
- Breathing or crying?
- Good muscle tone?
- Color pink?
- Term gestation?

No

- Provide warmth
- Position; clear airway*
  (as necessary)
- Dry, stimulate, reposition
- Give O₂ (as necessary)

- Evaluate respirations,
  heart rate, and color

30 SECONDS

Apnea   *or HR<100*

- Provide positive-pressure ventilation*

HR<60   *HR>60*

30 SECONDS

- Provide positive-pressure ventilation*
- Administer chest compressions

HR<60

- Administer
  epinephrine*   *HR<60*

*Endotracheal intubation may
be considered at several steps.

Recheck effectiveness of
- **Ventilation**
- **Chest compressions**
- **Endotracheal intubation**
- **Epinephrine delivery**
Consider possibility of
- **Hypovolemia**
- **Severe metabolic acidosis**

*HR<60 or persistent cyanosis
or failure to ventilate*   *HR absent*

Consider:
- **Airway malformations**
- **Lung problems, such as**
  – Pneumothorax
  – Diaphragmatic hernia
- **Congenital heart disease**

Consider discontinuing
resuscitation

What should you do if there is still no improvement?

If the baby has been severely compromised but all resuscitation efforts have gone smoothly, you should have reached the point of giving epinephrine relatively quickly. No more than 30 seconds each should be required for a trial of each of the following four steps of resuscitation —

- Assessment and initial steps
- Positive-pressure ventilation
- Positive-pressure ventilation and chest compressions
- Positive-pressure ventilation, chest compressions, and epinephrine

Endotracheal intubation also likely would have been performed. You would have checked the efficacy of each of the steps, and you would have considered the possibility of hypovolemia and/or metabolic acidosis.

If the heart rate is detectable but remains below 60 beats per minute, it is still likely that the baby will be able to be resuscitated, unless the baby is either extremely immature or has a lethal congenital malformation. If you are certain that ventilation, chest compressions, and medications are being delivered appropriately, you might then consider mechanical causes of poor response, such as an airway malformation, pneumothorax, diaphragmatic hernia, or congenital heart disease (discussed in Lesson 7).

If the heart rate is absent, or no progress is being made in certain conditions, such as extreme prematurity, it may be appropriate to discontinue resuscitative efforts. The ethical considerations of when to discontinue unsuccessful resuscitation efforts also will be discussed in Lesson 7.

Lesson 6 Review

(The answers are at the end of the lesson.)

1. Most babies who need resuscitation will respond to positive-pressure ventilation and chest compressions. However, a small number will have heart rates below 60 beats per minute after 90 seconds of resuscitation. Fewer than _____ babies per 1,000 births will need epinephrine to stimulate their hearts.

2. Ninety seconds into a resuscitation, the baby's heart rate is less than 60 beats per minute. You should now give _____ by the most quickly accessible route while continuing chest compressions and _____ .

3. Which drugs should NOT be administered through an endotracheal tube?
   ____ Epinephrine
   ____ Naloxone
   ____ Sodium bicarbonate

4. A newborn is intubated and is receiving positive-pressure ventilation and chest compressions. If you want to administer epinephrine quickly, which route should you choose?
   ____ Endotracheal tube
   ____ Umbilical vein

5. You may follow an injection of endotracheal epinephrine with an injection of _____ _____ to ensure that most of the drug is delivered to the baby and not left in the catheter or tube.

6. Epinephrine is a cardiac (stimulant) (depressant).

7. Epinephrine (increases) (decreases) the strength of cardiac contractions and (increases) (decreases) the rate of cardiac contractions.

8. The recommended concentration of epinephrine for newborns is (1:1,000) (1:10,000).

9. The recommended dose of epinephrine for newborns is _____ mL/kg of a 1:10,000 solution.

Lesson 6 Review — *continued*

(The answers are at the end of the lesson.)

10. Epinephrine should be given (slowly) (as quickly as possible).

11. What should you do approximately 30 seconds after giving epinephrine? _____

12. If the baby's heart rate remains below 60 beats per minute, you can repeat the dose of epinephrine every _____ to _____ minutes.

13. If the baby's heart rate remains below 60 beats per minute after you have given epinephrine, you also should check to make sure that ventilation is producing good chest movement and that _____ _____ are being done correctly.

14. If the baby is pale, there is evidence of blood loss, and resuscitation is not resulting in improvement, you should consider giving _____ mL/kg of _____ by _____ .

15. Two characteristics of sodium bicarbonate are hypertonicity and conversion to CO_2. These factors encourage what precautions when giving it during resuscitation?
    (1) _____
    (2) _____
    (3) _____

16. Which route of delivery is contraindicated for giving sodium bicarbonate during resuscitation? _____ .

Performance Checklist
Lesson 6 — Medications

Instructor: The learner should be instructed to talk through the procedure as it is demonstrated. Judge the performance of each step and check (✓) the box when the action is completed correctly. If done incorrectly, circle the box so that you can discuss that step later. You will need to provide information at several points concerning the condition of the baby.

Learner: To successfully complete this checklist, you should be able to perform all the steps and make all the correct decisions in the procedure. You should talk through the procedure as you perform it.

Equipment and Supplies

For epinephrine via endotracheal tube
Intubation manikin
Epinephrine 1:10,000 (or simulation)
1-mL syringes
Medication labels
Normal saline flush
5F feeding tube or catheter with connector to accomodate syringe (optional)
Self-inflating bag with reservoir or
Flow-inflating bag with oxygen source
Code sheet for recording medication

For epinephrine or volume expander via umbilical venous catheter
Umbilical cord segment for cannulation (simulated or real)*
3-mL syringes
20-mL syringes
3-way stopcock
3.5F or 5F umbilical catheters
Normal saline flush
Povidone-iodine applicator (or simulated)
Gloves
Umbilical tape
Scalpel handle and blade
Curved hemostat
Forceps
Epinephrine 1:10,000 (or simulation)
Normal saline for volume expansion (or simulation)
Needle
Medication labels
Code sheet for recording medication

* *If using human umbilical cord segments*
Human umbilical cord stabilized in bottle nipple (see instructor's manual)
Personal protection equipment (barrier gown, gloves, face protection)
Appropriate disposal supplies (laundry bag, sharps container, biohazard bag)
Waterproof pad for table surface
Handwashing facility

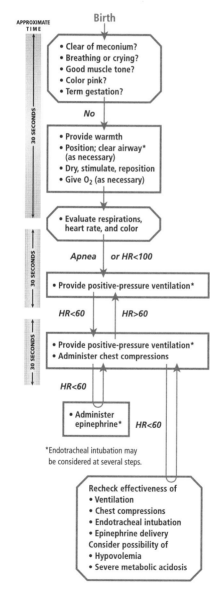

Performance Checklist
Lesson 6 — Medications

Name _____ Instructor _____ Date _____

The second part of this Performance Checklist is divided into two roles — inserting the catheter and preparing/administering medications. If only one learner is being evaluated, the learner may perform both roles or the instructor may take the role of the other person.

Instructor's statements are in quotes. Learner's questions and correct responses are in bold type. Instructor should check boxes as the learner answers correctly.

"A full-term newborn presented with poor muscle tone, apnea, and central cyanosis. She was placed under a radiant warmer. Resuscitation so far has included bag-and-mask ventilation, endotracheal intubation, and 30 seconds of chest compressions. The heart rate is still 30 bpm. Please demonstrate what you would do."

☐ **Asks for an estimate of baby's size**

"The baby appears to weigh about 3 kg."

☐ **States that epinephrine is required and correct dose**

☐ **Checks medication label for name of medication and concentration**

☐ **Uses proper-sized syringe (1mL)**

☐ **Calculates correct volume of epinephrine to be administered**

☐ **Draws up correct dose of epinephrine into 1-mL syringe and labels appropriately**

☐ **Prepares normal saline flush or dilutes epinephrine with saline to full volume of syringe and labels appropriately**

☐ **Double-checks medication and dose by verbalizing medication and dose to be administered**

☐ **Gives drug directly into the tube**
- **Does not deposit medication into connector**
- **Flushes with saline (unless drug pre-diluted)**

       OR

Gives drug through feeding tube or catheter
- **Inserts feeding tube or catheter down endotracheal tube**
- **Administers drug**
- **Flushes with saline (unless drug pre-diluted)**

☐ **Provides ventilation after drug is instilled**

☐ **Records medication, dose, route, time, and newborn response on code sheet**

"The heart rate remains less than 60 bpm and the baby appears very pale. A decision is made to administer a volume expander intravenously. Demonstrate what you would do."

Inserts   ## Prepares

☐ Specifies doses of medications needed

Prepares umbilical catheter for insertion

    Fills a 3-mL syringe with normal saline   ☐

    Attaches three-way stopcock to umbilical catheter   ☐

    Flushes umbilical catheter and stopcock with normal saline   ☐

    Closes the stopcock to the catheter to prevent loss of fluid and air entry into catheter   ☐

Prepares medications

    Draws up correct dose of isotonic crystalloid and labels syringe   ☐

    Draws up normal saline flush   ☐

☐ Preps the base and lower few centimeters of the cord with povidone-iodine

☐ Ties umbilical tape loosely around base of cord

☐ Using sterile technique, cuts cord with scalpel to expose vein

Positions umbilical venous catheter in umbilical vein

    ☐ Inserts catheter into vein

    Opens stopcock between baby and syringe and gently aspirates syringe to detect blood return   ☐

    ☐ Advances catheter until blood return is detected

    Clears any air from catheter and stopcock   ☐

Double-checks medication and dose by verbalizing medication and dose to be administered   ☐

☐ Holds catheter in place as drug or volume expander is administered with no air bubbles introduced   ☐

Flushes tubing to ensure proper dose   ☐

☐ Listens to chest and asks for heart rate and respirations

Records medication/volume expander, dose, route, time, and newborn response on code sheet   ☐

"You detect 12 beats in 6 seconds. Baby is still apneic."

Inserts   ## Prepares

☐ Indicates that chest compressions can stop, positive-pressure ventilation should continue, and catheter can be removed

☐ Removes catheter, secures umbilical tape, and monitors for bleeding at site

Overall

☐ Understands technique to withdraw single dose of drug from original packaging   ☐

☐ Understands directional use of stopcock   ☐

☐ Recognizes appropriate volume for drug or volume expander

☐ Administers drug or volume expander over appropriate periods of time   ☐

☐ Uses standard precautions and sterile technique

Key Points

1. Epinephrine, a cardiac stimulant, is indicated when the heart rate remains below 60 beats per minute, despite 30 seconds of assisted ventilation and another 30 seconds of coordinated chest compressions and ventilations.

2. Recommended epinephrine
   - Concentration: 1:10,000
   - Route: Endotracheal tube or intravenously
   - Dose: 0.1 to 0.3 mL/kg
   - Preparation: Correct dose of 1:10,000 solution in 1-mL syringe
   - Rate: *Rapidly* — as quickly as possible

3. Epinephrine may be given via endotracheal tube or umbilical vein; however, the endotracheal route is often faster and more accessible than placing an umbilical catheter.

4. Indications for volume expander include
   - Baby is not responding to resuscitation
   - Evidence of blood loss (pale color, weak pulses, persistently high or low heart rate, no improvement in circulatory status despite resuscitation efforts)

5. Recommended volume expander
   - Solution: Normal saline
   - Dose: 10 mL/kg
   - Route: Umbilical vein
   - Preparation: Correct volume drawn into large syringe
   - Rate: Over 5 to 10 minutes

6. Indication for sodium bicarbonate
   - Severe metabolic acidosis is suspected or is proven by blood gas analysis

7. Do not give sodium bicarbonate unless the lungs are being adequately ventilated.

8. Sodium bicarbonate is very caustic and should NOT be given through an endotracheal tube.

Key Points — *continued*

9. Recommended sodium bicarbonate

   - Solution: 4.2% (0.5 mEq/mL)

   - Dose: 2 mEq/kg (4 mL/kg of 4.2% solution)

   - Route: Umbilical vein, from which there is good blood return

   - Preparation: Correct volume of 0.5 mEq/mL (4.2%) solution in a 10-mL syringe

   - Rate: *Slowly* — no faster than 1mEq/kg/min

10. If the baby shows no improvement after administration of sodium bicarbonate, check for

    - Appropriate delivery of ventilation

    - Appropriate delivery of chest compressions

    - Appropriate delivery of medications

    - Mechanical causes of poor response, such as airway malformation, pneumothorax, diaphragmatic hernia, or congenital heart disease

Answers to Questions

1. Fewer than **two** babies per 1,000 births will need epinephrine to stimulate their hearts.

2. You should give **epinephrine** while continuing chest compressions and **ventilation**.

3. **Sodium bicarbonate** should not be administered though an endotracheal tube.

4. The **endotracheal tube** is the quickest route to administer epinephrine.

5. You should follow an injection of epinephrine with an injection of **normal saline**.

6. Epinephrine is a cardiac **stimulant**.

7. Epinephrine **increases** the strength of cardiac contractions and increases the rate of cardiac contractions.

8. The recommended concentration of epinephrine for newborns is **1:10,000**.

9. The recommended dose of epinephrine for newborns is **0.1 to 0.3** mL/kg of 1:10,000 solution.

10. Epinephrine should be given **as quickly as possible**.

11. You should **check the heart rate** approximately 30 seconds after giving epinephrine.

12. If the baby's heart rate remains below 60 beats per minute, you can repeat the dose of epinephrine every **3 to 5** minutes.

13. Check to make sure that ventilation is producing good chest movement and that **chest compressions** are being done correctly.

14. You should consider giving **10 mL/kg** of **normal saline** by **umbilical vein**.

15. Sodium bicarbonate should be given (1) **slowly**, (2) **with good ventilation**, and (3) **into a large vein**.

16. Sodium bicarbonate should not be given through the **endotracheal tube**.

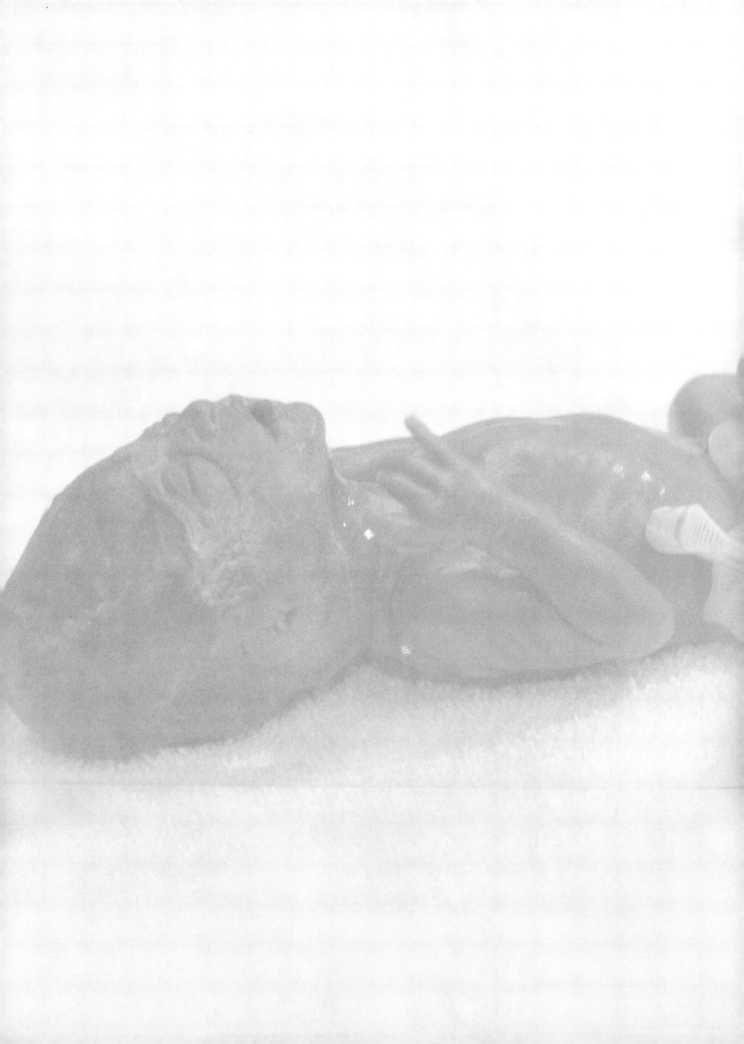

Special Considerations

In Lesson 7 you will learn

- Special situations that may complicate resuscitation and cause ongoing problems
- Subsequent management of the baby who has required resuscitation
- Ethical considerations about starting and stopping resuscitation
- How the principles in this program can be applied to babies who require resuscitation beyond the immediate newborn period or outside the hospital delivery room

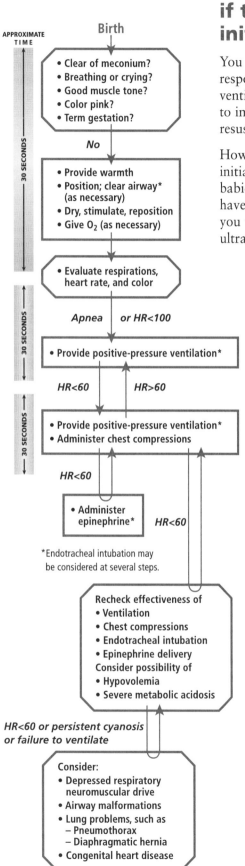

APPROXIMATE
TIME

Birth

30 SECONDS

- Clear of meconium?
- Breathing or crying?
- Good muscle tone?
- Color pink?
- Term gestation?

No

- Provide warmth
- Position; clear airway*
  (as necessary)
- Dry, stimulate, reposition
- Give O₂ (as necessary)

- Evaluate respirations,
  heart rate, and color

30 SECONDS

Apnea *or HR<100*

- Provide positive-pressure ventilation*

HR<60 *HR>60*

30 SECONDS

- Provide positive-pressure ventilation*
- Administer chest compressions

HR<60

- Administer
  epinephrine*

HR<60

*Endotracheal intubation may
be considered at several steps.

Recheck effectiveness of
- Ventilation
- Chest compressions
- Endotracheal intubation
- Epinephrine delivery
Consider possibility of
- Hypovolemia
- Severe metabolic acidosis

*HR<60 or persistent cyanosis
or failure to ventilate*

Consider:
- Depressed respiratory
  neuromuscular drive
- Airway malformations
- Lung problems, such as
  – Pneumothorax
  – Diaphragmatic hernia
- Congenital heart disease

What complications should you consider if the baby still is not doing well after initial attempts at resuscitation?

You have learned that nearly all compromised newborns will respond to appropriate stimulation and measures to improve ventilation. A few may require chest compressions and medications to improve; a very small number will die, despite all appropriate resuscitation measures.

However, there is another small group of newborns that will respond initially to resuscitation but then will remain compromised. These babies may have a congenital malformation or infection, or they may have suffered a complication of birth or of resuscitation. Sometimes you will know of the problem before birth as a result of antepartum ultrasound or some other method of antenatal diagnosis.

The continuing difficulty you encounter will be different for every baby, depending on the underlying problem. Some babies may fail to begin spontaneous breathing after you have given effective positive-pressure ventilation. You may be unable to ventilate other babies. Still other babies may be easily ventilated and may breathe easily but will remain cyanotic or have a low heart rate.

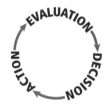

The most effective approach for babies who do not continue to improve after resuscitation will depend on their specific clinical presentation.

- Does the baby fail to begin spontaneous respirations?
- Does positive-pressure ventilation fail to result in adequate ventilation of the lungs?
- Does the baby remain cyanotic or bradycardic despite good ventilation?

Each of these three questions will be addressed separately.

What if the baby fails to begin spontaneous respirations?

If positive-pressure ventilation has resulted in the heart rate and color improving to normal but the baby still has poor muscle tone and fails to breathe spontaneously, the baby may have depressed brain or muscle activity from

- Brain injury (hypoxic-ischemic encephalopathy [HIE]) or a congenital neuromuscular disorder

or

- Sedation due to drugs previously administered to the mother and passed to the baby across the placenta

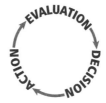 **Giving a narcotic antagonist is not the correct first therapy for a baby who is not breathing. The baby first should be given positive-pressure ventilation.**

Narcotics given to the mother to relieve pain associated with labor commonly inhibit respiratory drive and activity in the newborn. In such cases, administration of naloxone (a narcotic antagonist) to the newborn will reverse the effect of narcotics on the baby.

*The indications for giving **naloxone** to the baby require both of the following to be present:*

- Severe respiratory depression after positive-pressure ventilation has restored a normal heart rate and color

and

- A history of maternal narcotic administration within the past 4 hours

You should continue to administer positive-pressure ventilation until the baby is breathing normally. The duration of action of the narcotic often exceeds that of naloxone, necessitating repeated doses of naloxone. Therefore, the baby should be observed closely for recurrent respiratory depression, necessitating repeated doses of naloxone.

 Caution: Do not give naloxone to the newborn of a mother who is suspected of being addicted to narcotics or is on methadone maintenance. This may result in the newborn having severe seizures.

Other drugs given to the mother, such as magnesium sulfate or non-narcotic analgesics or general anesthetics, also can depress respirations in the newborn and will not respond to naloxone. If maternal narcotics were not given to the mother or if naloxone does not result in restoring spontaneous respirations, you should continue to administer positive-pressure ventilation and transport the baby to the nursery for further evaluation and management.

Naloxone Hydrochloride

Recommended concentration =
1.0 mg/mL solution

Recommended route =
Endotracheal or intravenous preferred;
intramuscular or subcutaneous
acceptable but delayed onset of action

Recommended dose =
0.1 mg/kg

What if positive-pressure ventilation fails to result in adequate ventilation of the lungs?

If you have cleared the airway, positioned the baby's head correctly in the "sniffing" position, ensured a tight seal between the mask and the baby's face, and used sufficient pressure when squeezing the resuscitation bag, you should see easy chest rise with each squeeze of the bag. Also, when you listen to the lungs with a stethoscope, you should hear good airflow in and out of the baby's lungs; heart rate, color, and tone should be improving. If you fail to see good chest movement and do not hear good airflow, one of the following may be the problem:

Mechanical blockage of the airway, such as from

• Meconium or mucus in the pharynx or trachea
• Choanal atresia
• Pharyngeal airway malformation (eg, Robin syndrome)
• Other rare conditions (eg, laryngeal web)

Impaired lung function, such as from

• Pneumothorax
• Congenital pleural effusions
• Congenital diaphragmatic hernia
• Pulmonary hypoplasia
• Extreme immaturity
• Congenital pneumonia

Mechanical blockage of the airway

Meconium or mucus blockage

Remember that the airway has not been tested until the time of birth. If initial suctioning of meconium or simple noninvasive measures, such as head positioning and suctioning the mouth and nose, fail to establish an adequate airway, you should consider suctioning the airway deeper in the mouth and nose with a large suction catheter (size 10F or 12F).

The surest way to rule out mucus or meconium in the airway is to insert an endotracheal tube and apply suction (as described in Lessons 2 and 5). Sometimes large plugs of meconium are blocking the airway of a meconium-stained baby.

Choanal atresia

The anatomy of a baby's airway requires the nasal airway to be patent for air to reach the lungs during spontaneous breathing. Babies cannot breathe easily through their mouths unless they are actively crying. Therefore, if the nasal airway is filled with mucus or meconium or if the nasal airway did not form properly (choanal atresia), the baby will be in severe respiratory distress (Figure 7.1).

You can test for choanal atresia by passing a small-caliber suction catheter into the posterior pharynx through one, and then the other, naris. Be sure to direct the catheter perpendicular to the baby's face so that it will travel along the floor of the nasal passageway. If the catheter will not pass when directed correctly, choanal atresia may be present. You will need to insert a plastic oral airway to allow air to pass through the mouth (Figure 7.2), or you may need to insert an endotracheal tube through the mouth.

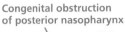
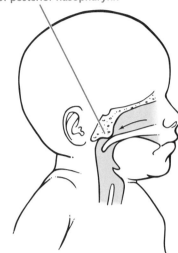

Figure 7.1. Choanal atresia

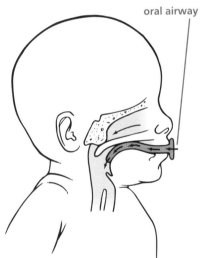

Figure 7.2. Oral airway for choanal atresia

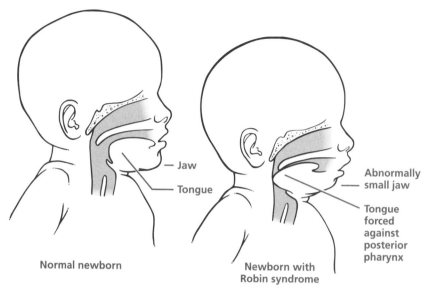

Figure 7.3. Normal newborn and newborn with Robin syndrome

Pharyngeal airway malformation (Robin syndrome)

Some babies are born with a very small mandible, which results in a critical narrowing of the pharyngeal airway (Figure 7.3). Over the next few months the mandible usually will grow to produce an adequate airway, but the baby may have considerable difficulty breathing after birth. The main problem is that the posteriorly placed tongue falls farther back into the pharynx and obstructs it just above the larynx.

Your first action should be to turn the baby on his stomach (prone). This often will allow the tongue to fall forward, thus opening the airway. If this is not successful, the next most effective means of achieving an airway for a baby with Robin syndrome is to insert a large catheter (12F) or small endotracheal tube (2.5 mm) through the nose, with the tip located deep in the posterior pharynx (Figure 7.4). This tube may relieve the suction that often causes the tongue to obstruct the airway. These two procedures (turning the baby prone and inserting a nasopharyngeal tube) usually will permit the baby to move air well on his own without the need for positive-pressure ventilation.

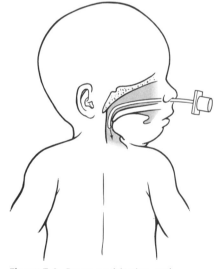

Figure 7.4. Prone positioning and placing a tube in posterior pharynx usually open the airway of a baby with Robin syndrome

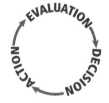

It usually is very difficult to place an endotracheal tube into the trachea of a baby with Robin syndrome. Prone positioning and a nasopharyngeal tube are often effective.

Other rare conditions

Congenital malformations, such as laryngeal webs, cystic hygroma, or congenital goiter, have been reported as rare causes of airway compromise in the newborn. Most, but not all, of these malformations will be evident by external examination of the baby. If an endotracheal tube cannot be passed, an emergency tracheostomy may be required.

Impaired lung function

Any substance that collects between the outside of the lung and the inside surface of the chest wall may prevent the lung from expanding within the chest. This will cause the baby to show signs of respiratory distress and perhaps to be persistently cyanotic and bradycardic.

Pneumothorax

It is not uncommon for small air leaks to develop in the airway as the lung of the newborn fills with air. The likelihood is increased significantly if positive-pressure ventilation is required, particularly in the presence of meconium or a lung malformation, such as congenital diaphragmatic hernia (see page 7-9). Air that leaks from inside the lung and collects in the pleural space is called a pneumothorax (Figure 7.5). If the pneumothorax becomes large enough, the trapped air under tension can prevent the lung from expanding and also can block blood flow to the lung, thus resulting in respiratory distress, cyanosis, and bradycardia.

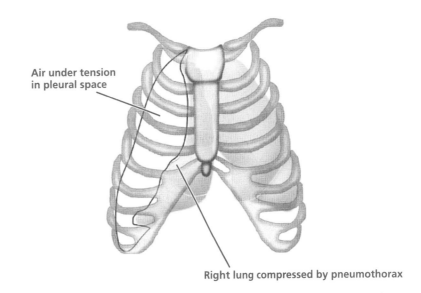

Air under tension in pleural space

Right lung compressed by pneumothorax

Figure 7.5. Pneumothorax compromising lung function

Breath sounds will be diminished on the side of the pneumothorax. Definitive diagnosis can be made with an x-ray. Transillumination of the chest may be helpful as a screening procedure.

Caution: Loss of breath sounds on the left also may be a reflection of the endotracheal tube being in too far.

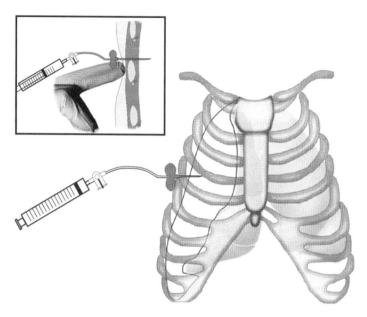

Figure 7.6. Decompression of pneumothorax or pleural effusion by needle inserted through 4th intercostal space into pleural space

If a pneumothorax causes significant respiratory distress, it should be relieved by placing a needle or chest tube into the pleural space (Figure 7.6).

Pleural effusions
Collections of fluid within the pleural space will cause the same symptoms as a pneumothorax. In rare circumstances, edema fluid, chyle (lymph fluid), or blood will collect in the pleural space of a newborn and prevent the lungs from adequately expanding. Usually, other signs of problems, such as total-body edema (hydrops fetalis), will be present in such newborns.

Diagnosis of fluid in the pleural space can be made by x-ray. If respiratory distress is significant, insert a needle or chest tube into the pleural space to drain the fluid.

The details of how to place a chest tube are beyond the scope of this program. However, in an emergency situation where the baby is in respiratory failure from a pneumothorax or pleural effusion, the air or fluid may be drained by needle aspiration. A small pneumothorax will absorb spontaneously and may not require treatment.

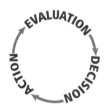

If a baby has worsening bradycardia and cyanosis and has asymmetric breath sounds after initially being resuscitated, you may decide to insert a needle into the chest on the side of the decreased breath sounds while waiting to obtain a chest x-ray.

A 21-gauge or 23-gauge butterfly needle should be inserted perpendicular to the chest wall and just over the top of the rib in the fourth intercostal space at the anterior axillary line on the suspected side. The fourth intercostal space is located at the level of the nipples. The butterfly needle is then connected to a three-way stopcock and 20-mL syringe. The stopcock is then opened between the syringe and the needle and the syringe is aspirated to remove air or fluid. When the syringe is full, the stopcock then may be closed to the chest while the syringe is emptied. The stopcock then may be reopened to the chest and more fluid or air aspirated until the baby's condition has improved. An x-ray then should be obtained to document the presence or absence of residual pneumothorax or effusion.

Congenital diaphragmatic hernia

The diaphragm normally separates the abdominal contents from the thoracic contents. When the diaphragm does not form completely, some of the abdominal contents (usually the intestines and the stomach, and sometimes the liver) enter the chest and prevent the lung on that side from developing normally. A diaphragmatic hernia often can be diagnosed by ultrasound before birth, although it may be completely unanticipated.

A baby with a diaphragmatic hernia will present with persistent respiratory distress and often will have an unusually flat appearing (scaphoid) abdomen, since the abdomen has less content than normal. Breath sounds will be diminished on the side of the hernia. These babies also have persistent pulmonary hypertension and, therefore, may remain persistently cyanotic from poor pulmonary blood flow.

When the baby is born, the underdeveloped lung cannot expand normally. If positive pressure is delivered by bag and mask during resuscitation, some of the oxygen enters the stomach and intestines (Figure 7.7). Since the intestines are in the chest, lung inflation is inhibited more. Also, positive pressure delivered to the underdeveloped lung may result in a pneumothorax.

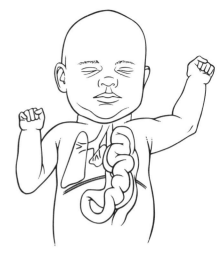

Figure 7.7. Compromised lung function from presence of a congenital diaphragmatic hernia

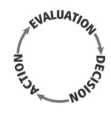

Babies with known or suspected diaphragmatic hernia should not receive prolonged resuscitation with bag and mask. They should have immediate endotracheal intubation, and a large orogastric catheter (10F) should be placed to evacuate the stomach contents (Figure 7.8).

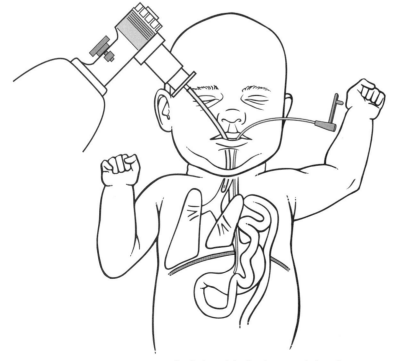

Figure 7.8. Stabilizing treatment for baby with diaphragmatic hernia (endotracheal tube in place and tube in stomach)

Pulmonary hypoplasia

Amniotic fluid must be present for the lungs to develop normally. Any condition that causes severe oligohydramnios (eg, renal agenesis) may result in pulmonary hypoplasia. Severe pulmonary hypoplasia usually is incompatible with survival.

Extreme immaturity

Babies with extremely immature lungs may be very difficult to ventilate, even with very high inflation pressures.

Congenital pneumonia

Although congenital pneumonia usually presents as worsening lung disease after birth, some overwhelming infections (eg, group B streptococcal disease) may present as respiratory failure at birth. Also, aspiration of amniotic fluid, particularly if contaminated with meconium, can cause severe respiratory compromise.

What if the baby remains cyanotic or bradycardic despite good ventilation?

First, ensure that the baby's chest is moving well, that there are good equal breath sounds on both sides of the chest, and that 100% oxygen is being given. If the baby still is bradycardic and/or cyanotic, he may have congenital heart disease. Confirmation with a chest x-ray, an electrocardiogram, and/or an echocardiogram may be necessary. However, remember that congenital heart block or even cyanotic congenital heart disease are rare conditions, while inadequate ventilation following birth is much more common.

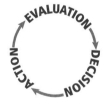

Babies with congenital heart disease are seldom critically ill immediately following birth. Problems with ventilation are almost always the cause of a failure to successfully resuscitate.

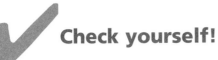 **Check yourself!**

(The answers are in the preceding section and at the end of the lesson.)

1. Babies who do not have spontaneous respirations and whose mothers have been given narcotic drugs should first receive _____ and then may be given _____.

2. Choanal atresia can be ruled out by what procedure? _____

3. Babies with Robin syndrome who have upper airway obstruction may be helped by placing a _____ and positioning them _____ . Endotracheal intubation of such babies is usually (easy) (difficult).

4. A pneumothorax or congenital diaphragmatic hernia should be considered if breath sounds are (equal) (unequal) on different sides of the chest.

5. You should suspect a congenital diaphragmatic hernia if the abdomen is _____ . Such babies should not be resuscitated with _____.

6. Persistent bradycardia and cyanosis during resuscitation most likely are caused by (lung problems) (heart problems).

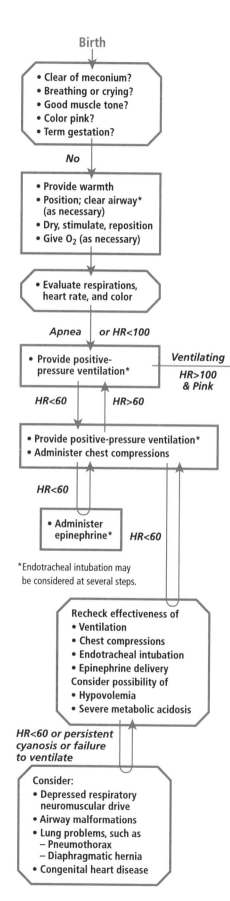

Birth

- Clear of meconium?
- Breathing or crying?
- Good muscle tone?
- Color pink?
- Term gestation?

No

- Provide warmth
- Position; clear airway* (as necessary)
- Dry, stimulate, reposition
- Give O₂ (as necessary)

- Evaluate respirations, heart rate, and color

Apnea | *or HR<100*

- Provide positive-pressure ventilation*

Ventilating
HR>100 & Pink → Ongoing care

HR<60 | *HR>60*

- Provide positive-pressure ventilation*
- Administer chest compressions

HR<60

- Administer epinephrine* | *HR<60*

*Endotracheal intubation may be considered at several steps.

Recheck effectiveness of
- Ventilation
- Chest compressions
- Endotracheal intubation
- Epinephrine delivery
Consider possibility of
- Hypovolemia
- Severe metabolic acidosis

HR<60 or persistent cyanosis or failure to ventilate

Consider:
- Depressed respiratory neuromuscular drive
- Airway malformations
- Lung problems, such as
  – Pneumothorax
  – Diaphragmatic hernia
- Congenital heart disease

What should you do after a baby has been successfully resuscitated?

Babies who have required substantial resuscitation have been severely stressed and are at risk for multi-organ damage that may not be immediately apparent.

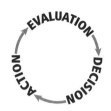

Do not assume that a baby who has been successfully resuscitated is healthy and can be treated as a routine newborn.

Some babies who have been resuscitated will be breathing spontaneously, while others still will require assisted ventilation. All should have a normal heart rate and be pink centrally. (There may be some acrocyanosis.)

If substantial resuscitation was required, the baby should be cared for in an environment where ongoing care can be provided. As was described in Lesson 1, ongoing care includes temperature management, close monitoring of vital signs, temperature control, and anticipation of complications. Continue to monitor oxygen saturation, heart rate, and blood pressure. Laboratory studies, such as hematocrit and blood glucose, should be obtained. Blood gas analysis may be indicated.

The likelihood of developing post-resuscitation complications will increase with the length and extent of resuscitation required. The pH and base deficit determined from cord blood or from blood drawn from the baby soon after resuscitation may be helpful in estimating the extent of compromise.

Common complications encountered in babies who have required resuscitation will be described next.

Pulmonary hypertension

As explained in Lesson 1, the blood vessels in the lungs are tightly constricted in the fetus. Ventilation and oxygenation at birth are the main stimuli that cause the blood vessels to relax, thus bringing blood to the lungs to pick up oxygen.

The pulmonary blood vessels in babies who have been extremely stressed at birth may remain constricted, thus resulting in cyanosis due to pulmonary hypertension. Severe pulmonary hypertension will result in further hypoxemia and may require tertiary-level therapies such as inhaled nitric oxide or extracorporeal membrane oxygenation (ECMO).

Additional pulmonary vasoconstriction may be prevented by avoiding episodes of hypoxemia after a baby has been resuscitated.

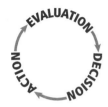

Use an oximeter and/or arterial blood gas determinations to be certain that a baby who required resuscitation remains well oxygenated.

Pneumonia and other lung complications

Babies who required resuscitation are at higher risk for developing pneumonia, either from aspiration syndrome or from a congenital infection that may have been responsible for causing the perinatal compromise. Neonatal pneumonia also is associated with pulmonary hypertension.

If a baby who required resuscitation continues to show any ongoing signs of respiratory distress or requirement for supplemental oxygen, consider evaluating the baby for pneumonia or bacterial sepsis and beginning parenteral antibiotics.

If acute respiratory deterioration occurs during or after resuscitation, consider the possibility that the baby may have developed a pneumothorax. Or, if the baby has remained intubated after resuscitation, consider that the tube may have become dislodged or become plugged with meconium or mucus.

Hypotension

Perinatal compromise can result in an insult to the heart muscle and/or to vascular tone. Heart murmurs often are audible from transient tricuspid insufficiency. If sepsis or blood loss was the reason that the baby required resuscitation, the effective circulating blood volume may be low.

Babies who required resuscitation should have heart rate and blood pressure monitoring until you are confident that blood pressure and peripheral perfusion are normal. Transfusion of blood or other volume expansion may be indicated, and some babies may require an infusion of an inotropic agent such as dopamine to assist cardiac output and vascular tone.

Fluid management

Perinatal compromise can result in renal dysfunction, which is usually transient (acute tubular necrosis) but can cause severe electrolyte and fluid shifts. Consider checking the urine for blood and protein to rule out acute tubular necrosis. Babies who have had cerebral hypoxia may also develop a syndrome of inappropriate antidiuretic hormone secretion (SIADH). Urine output, body weight, and serum electrolyte levels should be checked frequently for the first few days after birth. Some may need their fluid and electrolyte intakes restricted until renal function returns to normal or SIADH resolves. Supplemental calcium may be required. Electrolyte abnormalities will increase the risk of cardiac arrhythmias.

Seizures or apnea

Newborns who have perinatal compromise and undergo resuscitation may later manifest symptoms of hypoxic-ischemic encephalopathy (HIE). Initially, the baby may have depressed muscle tone, but after several hours seizures may appear. Apnea or hypoventilation may also be a reflection of hypoxic-ischemic encephalopathy. These same symptoms may also be a manifestation of metabolic or electrolyte disturbance, such as hypoglycemia, hyponatremia, or hypocalcemia.

Babies who have required extensive resuscitation should be monitored closely for seizures. Glucose, electrolyte, and/or anticonvulsant (eg, phenobarbital) therapy may be required.

Hypoglycemia

Metabolism under conditions of oxygen deprivation, which may occur during perinatal compromise, consumes much more glucose than the same metabolism occurring in the presence of oxygen. Although initially catecholamine secretion will cause serum glucose to be elevated, glucose stores (glycogen) become depleted rapidly during perinatal compromise and hypoglycemia may result. Glucose is essential for normal brain function in newborns.

Babies who required resuscitation should have their blood sugar levels checked soon after resuscitation and then sequentially, until several values have been within normal limits and adequate glucose intake has been ensured. Intravenous glucose will often be necessary to treat hypoglycemia.

Feeding problems

The gastrointestinal tract of a newborn is very sensitive to hypoxia-ischemia. Ileus, gastrointestinal bleeding, and even necrotizing enterocolitis can result. Also, because of neurologic insult, sucking patterns and coordination of sucking, swallowing, and breathing may take several days to recover. Intravenous fluids and nutrition may be required during this time.

Temperature management

Babies who have been resuscitated may become cold for a variety of reasons. Ongoing studies are examining whether cooling may be helpful for babies who have hypoxic-ischemic encephalopathy. Until this research is complete, maintaining a normal body temperature is advised.

 Hyperthermia can be very injurious to a baby. Be careful not to overheat the baby during or following resuscitation.

Babies' temperatures should be maintained in the normal range.

PREMATURITY POINTERS

Premature babies who required resuscitation are at risk for all of the post-resuscitation complications listed previously. However, the following issues are of particular concern:

- *Temperature management: Small babies tend to lose heat quickly. Premature babies who have required resuscitation should have their temperatures checked upon arrival to the nursery.*

- *Immature lungs: Babies born significantly preterm are likely to develop respiratory distress syndrome from surfactant deficiency. They may require endotracheal intubation soon after birth for ventilatory assistance and/or for administration of surfactant.*

- *Intracranial hemorrhage: Premature babies have a fragile germinal matrix in their brains. Resuscitation-associated hypoxic-ischemic encephalopathy, rapid changes in vascular volume, or unnecessarily rough handling during cardiopulmonary resuscitation may be associated with germinal matrix hemorrhage.*

- *Hypoglycemia: Preterm babies have fewer glycogen stores. Therefore, the hypoglycemia that is often associated with perinatal compromise is even more likely to occur in premature babies.*

- *Necrotizing enterocolitis: Premature babies who have had perinatal compromise are at particularly high risk for severe bowel injury (necrotizing enterocolitis). The more immature the baby, the greater the risk. Feedings should be introduced slowly.*

- *Oxygen injury: Premature babies are very sensitive to high arterial oxygen tension. Therefore, their oxygen levels should be kept in a normal range after resuscitation.*

Post-Resuscitation Care

Organ System	Potential Complication	Post-Resuscitation Action
Brain	Apnea Seizures	Monitor for apnea Support ventilation as needed Monitor glucose and electrolytes Avoid hyperthermia Consider anticonvulsant therapy
Lungs	Pulmonary hypertension Pneumonia Pneumothorax Transient tachypnea Meconium aspiration syndrome Surfactant deficiency	Maintain adequate oxygenation and ventilation Consider antibiotics Obtain x-ray if respiratory distress Consider surfactant therapy Delay feedings if respiratory distress
Cardiovascular	Hypotension	Monitor blood pressure and heart rate Consider inotrope (eg, dopamine) and/or volume replacement
Kidneys	Acute tubular necrosis	Monitor urine output Restrict fluids if oliguric volume and vascular volume are adequate Monitor serum electrolytes
Gastrointestinal	Ileus Necrotizing enterocolitis	Delay initiation of feedings Give intravenous fluids Consider parenteral nutrition
Metabolic/ Hematologic	Hypoglycemia Hypocalcemia; hyponatremia Anemia Thrombocytopenia	Monitor blood sugar Monitor electrolytes Monitor hematocrit Monitor platelets

✔ Check yourself!

(The answers are in the preceding section and at the end of the lesson.)

7. After resuscitation of a newborn, blood pressure in the pulmonary circuit is more likely to be (high) (low). Adequate oxygenation is likely to cause the pulmonary blood flow to (increase) (decrease).

8. If a meconium-stained baby has been resuscitated and then develops acute deterioration, a _____ should be suspected.

9. A baby who required resuscitation still has low blood pressure and poor perfusion after having been given a blood transfusion for suspected perinatal blood loss. He may require an infusion of _____ to improve his cardiac output and vascular tone.

10. Babies who have been resuscitated may have suffered kidney damage and are more likely to need (more) (less) fluids after the resuscitation.

11. A baby has a seizure 10 hours after being resuscitated. A blood sugar screen and serum electrolytes are normal. What class of drug should be used to treat her seizure? _____

12. List three causes of seizures following resuscitation.
    (1) _____
    (2) _____
    (3) _____

13. Because energy stores are consumed faster in the absence of oxygen, blood _____ levels may be low following resuscitation.

What ethical principles should be used in deciding when to start and when to stop neonatal resuscitation?

Many health care workers and parents are concerned that survivors of a prolonged resuscitation are likely to have severe disability. The following ethical guidelines may be useful:

- The ethical principles regarding resuscitation of newborns should be no different from those followed in resuscitating an older child or adult.

- In general, there is no advantage to delayed, graded, or partial resuscitation and support. If the newborn survives, outcome may be worsened as a result of this approach.

- There is no ethical mandate that prohibits withdrawal of support once it has been initiated.

- Try to base decisions about withdrawal or noninitiation of resuscitation on as much objective information as possible. Since much of the needed information often is unavailable at the time of delivery (eg, ultrasound scanning of the baby, subspecialist evaluation), resuscitation efforts frequently will continue for longer in the delivery area than later in the newborn period.

- Whenever the possibility of resuscitation can be anticipated, make every effort to discuss it with the family before delivery.

Are there situations in which noninitiation of resuscitation is reasonable?

The delivery of extremely immature babies and those with severe congenital anomalies raises questions about initiation of resuscitation. Noninitiation of resuscitation in the delivery room is appropriate for conditions such as

- Newborns with confirmed gestation of less than 23 weeks or birthweight less than 400 g*
- Anencephaly
- Babies with confirmed trisomy 13 or 18

Current data support that resuscitation of these newborns is very likely to result in non-survival or survival with severe disability.

However, be cautious about predetermining your resuscitation efforts before the baby is born based on predicted gestational age or birthweight.

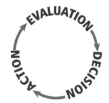 **The usual techniques used for obstetrical dating are accurate only to ± 1 to 2 weeks. Before deciding not to resuscitate, antenatal predictions should be confirmed by your examination of the baby.**

*Note: The limits of viability have undergone considerable change over the past 30 years. It is anticipated that this change will continue.

What should you do if your examination of the baby immediately after birth leaves you uncertain as to the chances of survival?

In cases of uncertain prognosis, including uncertain gestational age, resuscitation options include a trial of therapy, noninitiation, or discontinuation of resuscitation following assessment of the baby. If doubt still exists after assessment, initial resuscitation and provision of life support will allow you time to gather more complete clinical information and to permit more input from the family. Withdrawal of support following collection of such data and discussion with the parents may then be appropriate. You should try to avoid a scenario where a decision is initially made not to resuscitate and then the decision changed to aggressively resuscitate many minutes later.

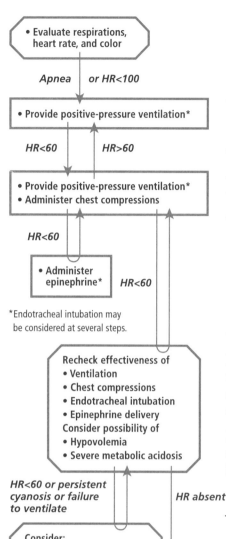

- Evaluate respirations, heart rate, and color

Apnea or *HR<100*

- Provide positive-pressure ventilation*

HR<60 *HR>60*

- Provide positive-pressure ventilation*
- Administer chest compressions

HR<60

- Administer epinephrine*

HR<60

*Endotracheal intubation may be considered at several steps.

Recheck effectiveness of
- Ventilation
- Chest compressions
- Endotracheal intubation
- Epinephrine delivery
Consider possibility of
- Hypovolemia
- Severe metabolic acidosis

HR<60 or persistent cyanosis or failure to ventilate

HR absent

Consider:
- Depressed respiratory neuromuscular drive
- Airway malformations
- Lung problems, such as
  – Pneumothorax
  – Diaphragmatic hernia
- Congenital heart disease

Consider discontinuing resuscitation

How long after there is no response is it appropriate to stop resuscitation efforts?

Discontinuation of resuscitation efforts may be appropriate after 15 minutes of absent heart rate in spite of complete and adequate resuscitation efforts. Current data support that resuscitation of newborns after 10 minutes of asystole is very unlikely to result in survival or survival without severe disability.

The lower portion of the resuscitation flow diagram is shown at the left with the "Consider discontinuing resuscitation" block at the bottom.

You have learned through the course of this program all of the essential steps required to resuscitate a severely depressed baby.

- Establishing an airway
- Delivering positive-pressure ventilation
- Administering chest compressions
- Administering epinephrine

If these four steps have been conducted well and you still have failed to resuscitate the baby, you have learned to consider other more rare causes of newborn compromise, such as congenital airway malformations or congenital heart disease.

If, after all of these steps and considerations, heart rate remains absent after 15 minutes, discontinuation of resuscitation efforts may be appropriate.

What role should the parents play in decisions about resuscitation?

Parents clearly should have a major role in determining the care delivered to their newborn. Before delivery you should make every effort to discuss with the parents your expectations about the baby's viability and the resuscitation approach that you intend to implement. However, informed consent should be based on as much information as possible, and the information that you will need to guide your actions may not be available until after delivery and perhaps until several hours after birth.

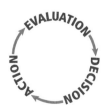

Caution: Be careful not to make promises about withholding or initiating resuscitation before the data needed to make that decision are available.

Are the resuscitation techniques different for babies born outside the hospital or beyond the immediate newborn period?

Throughout this program, you have learned about resuscitating newly born babies who were born in the hospital and were having difficulty making the transition from intrauterine to extrauterine life. Some babies, of course, may encounter difficulty and require resuscitation after being born outside of the hospital, and other babies will require resuscitation beyond the immediate newborn period.

Some examples of babies who may require resuscitation under different circumstances include

- A baby who delivers precipitously at home or in a motor vehicle
- A baby who develops apnea in the nursery
- A 2-week-old baby with sepsis who presents to the doctor's office in shock
- An intubated baby in the neonatal intensive care unit who deteriorates acutely

While the event precipitating the need for resuscitation may be different, the physiologic principles and the steps you should take to restore vital signs during the newborn period (first month after birth) remain the same.

- Warm, position, clear airway, stimulate the baby to breathe, and give oxygen (as necessary).
- Establish effective ventilation.
- Provide chest compressions.
- Administer medications.

 The priority for resuscitating babies at any time during the newborn period, regardless of location, should be to restore adequate ventilation.

Once you have ensured that ventilation is adequate, you should consider information that may be available about the baby's history in guiding the focus of your resuscitation efforts.

Although this program was not designed to teach neonatal resuscitation in these other venues, some strategies for applying the principles outside the delivery room will be presented in the next few pages. More details are available through other programs, such as the Pediatric Advanced Life Support (PALS) program of the American Heart Association or the Pediatric Education for Prehospital Professionals (PEPP) program of the American Academy of Pediatrics.

Case 6. Resuscitation of an apparently normal newborn

A baby weighing 3,400 g is born in the hospital at term after an uncomplicated pregnancy, labor, and delivery. The transitional period is uneventful; he remains with his mother and begins breastfeeding soon after birth.

At approximately 20 hours of age he is found by his mother to be apneic and unresponsive in his bassinet. She activates the emergency alarm, and a perinatal nurse on the floor responds immediately.

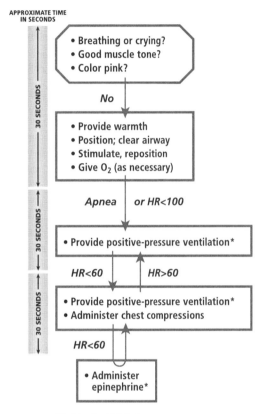

APPROXIMATE TIME
IN SECONDS

30 SECONDS

- Breathing or crying?
- Good muscle tone?
- Color pink?

No

- Provide warmth
- Position; clear airway
- Stimulate, reposition
- Give O₂ (as necessary)

Apnea or HR<100

30 SECONDS

- Provide positive-pressure ventilation*

HR<60   *HR>60*

30 SECONDS

- Provide positive-pressure ventilation*
- Administer chest compressions

HR<60

- Administer epinephrine*

*Endotracheal intubation may be considered at several steps.

The baby is found to be apneic, limp, and blue. He is placed under a radiant warmer, and his airway is opened by placing his head in the "sniffing" position and by suctioning his mouth and nose with a bulb syringe. He still does not resume breathing after having his back rubbed and the soles of his feet flicked. The nurse calls for help.

A self-inflating resuscitation bag and mask is readily available and is used to deliver positive-pressure ventilation. A second nurse arrives to help and attaches the bag to 100% oxygen. After approximately 30 seconds of positive-pressure ventilation, the second nurse uses a stethoscope to check the heart rate and finds it to be 30 beats per minute (bpm).

Chest compressions are started and coordinated with positive-pressure ventilation. After 30 seconds the heart rate is checked again and found to be 40 bpm. A third clinician arrives and inserts an endotracheal tube. One milliliter of 1:10,000 epinephrine is administered into the endotracheal tube. After another 30 seconds, the heart rate is found to be 80 bpm.

Chest compressions are discontinued, and positive-pressure ventilation is continued. After another minute, the heart rate increases to more than 100 bpm, and the baby begins breathing spontaneously.

The baby is connected to a pulse oximeter and is transferred to a transport incubator. He is moved to the nursery for evaluation of the cause of his respiratory arrest.

What are some of the different strategies needed to resuscitate outside the hospital or beyond the immediate newborn period?

Temperature control

Maintaining normal body temperature during resuscitation remains an important concept, but it becomes less difficult if the baby is not newly born, since the baby generally will not be wet. If the baby is newly born and requires resuscitation outside of the hospital, maintaining body temperature may become a major challenge, because you likely will not have a radiant warmer readily available. Some suggestions for minimizing heat loss are as follows:

• Turn up the heat source in the room or vehicle.

• Dry the baby well with bath towels, a blanket, or clean clothing.

• Use the mother's body as a heat source. Consider placing the baby skin-to-skin on the mother's chest and covering both baby and mother with a blanket.

Clearing the airway

If resuscitation is required outside a delivery room or nursery, vacuum suction will often not be readily available. Suggestions for methods of clearing the airway are as follows:

• Use a bulb syringe.

• Wipe the mouth and nose with a clean handkerchief or other cloth wrapped around your index finger.

Ventilation

Babies born outside the hospital may still require positive-pressure ventilation to ventilate the lungs. If a resuscitation bag-and-mask device is unavailable, positive-pressure ventilation can be delivered by mouth-to-mouth-and-nose. The baby should be placed in the "sniffing" position, and the resuscitator's mouth should make a tight seal over the baby's mouth and nose. With particularly large babies or small-mouthed resuscitators, it may be necessary to cover only the baby's mouth with the resuscitator's mouth while the baby's nose is pinched to seal the airway. There is a risk of transmission of infectious disease with this technique.

Vascular access

Catheterization of the umbilical vessels is generally not an option outside the hospital or beyond the first several days after birth. In such cases, prompt cannulation of a peripheral vein or insertion of an intraosseus needle into the tibia are reasonable alternatives. Detailed description of these techniques is beyond the scope of this program.

Medications

Epinephrine should still be the primary drug used for resuscitation of babies who do not respond to positive-pressure ventilation and chest compressions. However, other medications (eg, calcium, adenosine) also may be necessary, depending on the cause of the arrest. The diagnostic steps required and the details of using these drugs are beyond the scope of this program.

Check yourself!

(The answers are in the preceding section and at the end of the lesson.)

14. List three conditions in which noninitiation of resuscitation is appropriate.
    (1) _____
    (2) _____
    (3) _____

15. It is reasonable to discontinue resuscitation efforts if a heart rate has been absent for _____ minutes.

16. You are likely to have (more) (less) (about the same) difficulty controlling body temperature of babies requiring resuscitation beyond the immediate newborn period.

17. The priority for resuscitating babies beyond the immediate newborn period should be to
    A. Defibrillate the heart
    B. Expand blood volume
    C. Establish effective ventilation
    D. Administer epinephrine
    E. Deliver chest compressions

18. If vacuum suction is not available to clear the airway, two alternative methods are _____ and _____.

19. If a 15-day-old baby requiring resuscitation had blood loss, vascular access routes include _____ and _____.

Will resuscitation of newborns as described in this textbook result in improved outcomes?

Birth asphyxia accounts for nearly 1 million deaths each year worldwide. Experience over the last century has shown that perinatal mortality can be reduced by more than 80% by improved obstetrical and newborn care.

Although resuscitation of children beyond the immediate newborn period is often unsuccessful, resuscitation at birth is usually successful. Studies have shown that term babies who appear to be recently stillborn have a greater than two-thirds likelihood of responding to resuscitation and surviving. Over two-thirds of those survivors were normal when evaluated during early childhood. While the information available on resuscitation of extremely preterm babies (less than 1,000 g birthweight) is somewhat less optimistic, they too have been shown to have a greater than 50% chance of survival, and the majority will have normal development if they survive.

Survival, of course, is not the only consideration. The physical and developmental potential of a baby's life can be profoundly affected by an insult experienced at birth. By helping the baby to make a smooth transition from intrauterine to extrauterine life, you can play a major role in providing the opportunity of a lifetime!

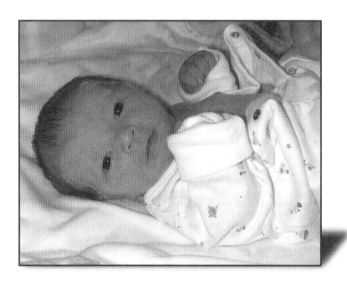

Lesson 7 Review

(The answers are at the end of the lesson.)

1. Babies who do not have spontaneous respirations and whose mothers have been given narcotics should first receive _____ and then may be given _____ .

2. Choanal atresia can be ruled out by what procedure? _____

3. Babies with Robin syndrome who have upper airway obstruction may be helped by placing a _____ and positioning them _____ . Endotracheal intubation of such babies is usually (easy) (difficult).

4. A pneumothorax or congenital diaphragmatic hernia should be considered if breath sounds are (equal) (unequal) on different sides of the chest.

5. You should suspect a congenital diaphragmatic hernia if the abdomen is _____ . Such babies should not be resuscitated with _____ .

6. Persistent bradycardia and cyanosis during resuscitation most likely are caused by (lung problems) (heart problems).

7. After resuscitation of a newborn, blood pressure in the pulmonary circuit is more likely to be (high) (low). Adequate oxygenation is likely to cause the pulmonary blood flow to (increase) (decrease).

8. If a meconium-stained baby has been resuscitated and then develops acute deterioration, a _____ should be suspected.

9. A baby who required resuscitation still has low blood pressure and poor perfusion after having been given a blood transfusion for suspected perinatal blood loss. He may require an infusion of _____ to improve his cardiac output and vascular tone.

Lesson 7 Review — *continued*

(The answers are at the end of the lesson.)

10. Babies who have been resuscitated may have suffered kidney damage and are more likely to need (more) (less) fluids after the resuscitation.

11. A baby has a seizure 10 hours after being resuscitated. A blood sugar screen and serum electrolytes are normal. What class of drug should be used to treat her seizure?

    _____

12. List three causes of seizures following resuscitation.
    (1) _____
    (2) _____
    (3) _____

13. Because energy stores are consumed faster in the absence of oxygen, blood _____ levels may be low following resuscitation.

14. List three conditions in which noninitiation of resuscitation is appropriate.
    (1) _____
    (2) _____
    (3) _____

15. It is reasonable to discontinue resuscitation efforts if a heart rate has been absent for _____ minutes.

16. You are likely to have (more) (less) (about the same) difficulty controlling body temperature of babies requiring resuscitation beyond the immediate newborn period.

17. The priority for resuscitating babies beyond the immediate newborn period should be to
    A. Defibrillate the heart
    B. Expand blood volume
    C. Establish effective ventilation
    D. Administer epinephrine
    E. Deliver chest compressions

Lesson 7 Review — *continued*

(The answers are at the end of the lesson.)

18. If vacuum suction is not available to clear the airway, two alternative methods are _____ and _____.

19. If a 15-day-old baby requiring resuscitation had blood loss, vascular access routes include _____ and _____.

Key Points

1. Reasons for failure to breathe after resuscitation include brain injury or a congenital neuromuscular disorder or sedatives recently given to the mother.

2. Naloxone given to the baby will counteract the respiratory depressant effects of narcotics previously given to the mother during labor. However, do not give naloxone if the mother is on methadone maintenance or is suspected of being addicted to narcotics.

3. Some reasons for a blocked airway include mucus/meconium, choanal atresia, and Robin syndrome.

4. Some reasons for failure of a lung to expand include pneumothorax, pleural effusions, diaphragmatic hernia, pulmonary hypoplasia, congenital pneumonia, and extreme immaturity.

5. Symptoms from choanal atresia can be helped by placing an oral airway.

6. Airway obstruction from Robin syndrome can be helped by inserting a nasopharyngeal tube and placing the baby prone.

7. In an emergency, a pneumothorax can be detected by transillumination and treated by inserting a needle in the chest.

8. If diaphragmatic hernia is suspected, avoid bag-and-mask resuscitation. Immediately intubate the trachea and insert an orogastric tube.

9. Persistent cyanosis and bradycardia are rarely caused by congenital heart disease.

10. A baby who has required resuscitation must have close monitoring and management of oxygenation, infection, blood pressure, fluids, apnea, blood sugar, feeding, and temperature.

11. Be careful not to overheat the baby during or following resuscitation.

12. Newborns should be treated by the same ethical principles that apply to treatment of adults and children.

13. Withdrawal of support after resuscitation may be ethical.

14. There are some conditions where noninitiation of resuscitation in the delivery room is appropriate.

15. Discontinuation of resuscitation is appropriate after 15 minutes of absent heart rate after complete and adequate resuscitation efforts have been attempted.

16. Restoring adequate ventilation remains the priority when resuscitating babies at birth in the delivery room or later in the nursery or other location.

Key Points — *continued*

17. Some alternative techniques for resuscitation outside of the delivery room include the following:

    • Maintain temperature by placing the baby skin-to-skin with the mother and raising the environmental temperature.

    • Clear airway with a bulb syringe or cloth on your finger.

    • Consider mouth-to-mouth-and-nose for administering positive pressure.

    • Cannulation of a peripheral vein or intraosseous space can be used for vascular access.

    • Medications other than or in addition to epinephrine may be needed, depending on the cause of the arrest.

18. Resuscitation of newborns after birth carries a better prognosis than resuscitation of older children or adults.

19. Immediate resuscitation of newborns usually results in their survival and normal development.

Answers to Questions

1. Babies whose respirations are depressed from maternal narcotics should first receive **positive-pressure ventilation** and then may be given **naloxone.**

2. Choanal atresia can be ruled out by **passing a nasopharyngeal catheter through the nares.**

3. Babies with Robin syndrome who have upper airway obstruction may be helped by placing a **nasopharyngeal tube** and positioning them **on their abdomens (prone)**. Endotracheal intubation of such babies is usually **difficult.**

4. A pneumothorax or congenital diaphragmatic hernia should be considered if breath sounds are **unequal** on different sides of the chest. If the trachea has been intubated, you also should check to be sure that the tube is not in too far.

5. You should suspect a congenital diaphragmatic hernia if the abdomen is **flat-appearing (scaphoid)**. Such babies should not be resuscitated with **bag and mask.**

6. Persistent bradycardia and cyanosis during resuscitation most likely are caused by **lung problems.**

7. After resuscitation of a newborn, blood pressure in the pulmonary circuit is more likely to be **high**. Adequate oxygenation is likely to cause the pulmonary vascular resistance to fall, and thus blood flow to **increase.**

8. If a meconium-stained baby has been resuscitated and then develops acute deterioration, a **pneumothorax** should be suspected. (An endotracheal tube plugged with meconium is also a consideration.)

9. The baby may require an infusion of **dopamine (or other inotrope)** to improve his cardiac output and vascular tone.

10. Babies who have been resuscitated are more likely to need **less** fluids after the resuscitation.

11. A baby with a seizure 10 hours after being resuscitated and with a normal blood sugar should be treated with **an anticonvulsant (eg, phenobarbital).**

12. Seizures following resuscitation may be caused by (1) **electrolyte abnormalities,** (2) **hypoxic-ischemic encephalopathy,** or (3) **hypoglycemia.**

13. Blood **sugar (glucose)** levels may be low following resuscitation.

14. Noninitiation of resuscitation is appropriate in any of the following situations: (1) **confirmed gestation less than 23 weeks** or **birthweight less than 400 g,** (2) **anencephaly,** (3) **confirmed trisomy 13 or 18.**

15. It is reasonable to discontinue resuscitation efforts if a heart rate has been absent for **15 minutes.**

Answers to Questions — *continued*

16. You are likely to have **less** difficulty controlling body temperature of babies requiring resuscitation beyond the immediate newborn period, since they usually will not be wet.

17. The priority for resuscitating babies beyond the immediate newborn period should be to **establish effective ventilation.**

18. If vacuum suction is not available to clear the airway, two alternative methods are **bulb suction** and **wiping the airway with a clean cloth.**

19. If a 15-day-old baby requiring resuscitation had blood loss, vascular access routes include **cannulation of a peripheral vein** and **insertion of an intraosseus needle.**

Performance Checklist
Megacode

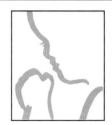

Instructor: This performance checklist is divided into 2 sections. All learners should complete part A. Have the learner complete Section B depending on the role that is most consistent with his or her clinical responsibilities. Factors to consider are

- Is the learner authorized to perform endotracheal intubation?
- Is the learner authorized to administer medications?

A learner responsible for performing none of the above should complete only Part A, but could also participate as Learner #2 in Part B.

Both sections will require more than one person. If only one learner is being evaluated, then you will need to serve as the other person(s). However, evaluating several people at once also will help to judge their ability to function as a team. The learner should be instructed to talk through the procedure as it is demonstrated. Judge the performance of each step and check (✓) the box when the action is completed correctly. If done incorrectly, circle the box so that you can discuss that step later. You will need to provide information at several points concerning the condition of the baby.

Learner: To successfully complete this checklist, you should be able to perform all the steps and make all the correct decisions in the procedure. You should talk through the procedure as you perform it.

Equipment and Supplies

Newborn resuscitation manikin
Intubation manikin
Radiant warmer or table to simulate warmer
Gloves (or may simulate this)
Stethoscope
Self-inflating bag with oxygen reservoir
or
Flow-inflating bag with pressure manometer and oxygen source
Larynogoscope with fresh batteries and functioning light source
Blade, No. 1 (term) for use with manikin or No. 0 if appropriate
ET tubes, 2.5, 3.0, 3.5, 4.0 mm
Stylet (optional)
Tape or ET tube securing device

Scissors (optional)
Suction device — suction setup with 10F or larger suction catheter
CO_2 detector (optional)
Meconium aspirator
Oral airway, premature and infant sizes
Clock with a second hand
Epinephrine 1:10,000 (or simulation)
1 mL syringes
Medication labels
Normal saline flush
5F feeding tube or catheter with connector to accommodate syringe (optional)
Code sheet for recording resuscitation activities

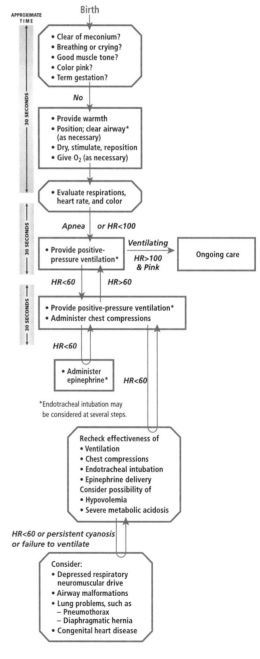

Performance Checklist
Megacode — Part A

Name _____ Instructor _____ Date _____

All participants should complete part A of this Performance Checklist. Responsibilities are described for two learners: one who ventilates and one who provides chest compressions. The location of the check box indicates which learner is responsible for each activity. Each learner may be asked to demonstrate skills in each role.

Instructor's statements are in quotes. Learner's questions and correct responses are in bold type. Instructor should check boxes as the learner answers correctly.

"A 37-year-old primiparous woman is admitted to the obstetrical floor in active labor at 38 weeks. The membranes ruptured 2 days ago. Fetal monitoring discloses a non-reassuring fetal heart rate pattern that is unresponsive to maternal positioning and oxygen administration. A decision is made to perform a cesarean section. How would you prepare for the baby's birth?"

☐ Requests extra personnel to be present for delivery
☐ Indicates use of standard precautions as appropriate to local regulations
☐ Locates and checks function of stethoscope

Warm
☐ Turns on radiant warmer
☐ Ensures availability of warm linen/towels

Position; clear airway
☐ Ensures availability of shoulder roll
☐ Locates bulb syringe
☐ Locates meconium aspirator device
☐ Ensures function of mechanical suction device with vacuum set at 100 mm Hg

Oxygenate and Ventilate
☐ Ensures presence and function of equipment for free-flow oxygen.
☐ Ensures that oxygen tubing is attached to flowmeter and bag.
☐ Turns on flowmeter to 5 L/min.
☐ If self-inflating bag used,
  • Ensures that reservoir is attached.
  • Checks function of valve assembly and pressure release valve.
☐ Checks function of oxygen bag by creating seal with mask against palm of hand. When bag inflates, desired pressure is created.
☐ Checks function of pressure manometer on flow-inflating bag (optional on self-inflating bag).

☐ If bag is not working properly, obtains and tests another.
☐ Locates laryngoscope and blade size 1 (term).
☐ Ensures bright light in laryngoscope.
☐ Locates various sizes endotracheal tubes.
☐ Locates and prepares stylet (optional).
☐ Locates tape or endotracheal tube securing device.
☐ Locates scissors.

Medicate
☐ Checks expiration date and concentration of 1:10,000 epinephrine
☐ Locates syringes and supplies necessary for desired instillation method of epinephrine
☐ Locates and checks expiration dates and concentrations of additional medications
  • Normal saline
  • Supplies for emergency umbilical venous catheter placement
  • 4.2% sodium bicarbonate
☐ Locates medication labels and waterproof marker
☐ Locates code sheet for recording activities

"At delivery the baby is limp and unresponsive. He is immediately handed to you. Demonstrate and explain what you would do. You may ask me about specific details of the baby's condition."

Learner #1   **Learner #2**

☐ *Is meconium present?*

"No, there is no meconium present."

☐ *Is the baby breathing or crying?*
☐ *Is there good muscle tone?*
☐ *Is the baby pink?*
☐ *Is the baby term?*

"The baby appears to be term. He had a few weak breaths, but has poor tone and is not yet pink."

This baby requires the initial steps of resuscitation.
☐ Places baby on preheated radiant warmer with neck slightly extended
☐ Suctions mouth, then nose
☐ Dries body and head
☐ Removes wet linen
☐ Repositions baby with neck slightly extended
☐ Administers oxygen as necessary

☐ Counts heart rate by palpating the cord or auscultating the chest for 6 seconds.
☐ *Is the baby breathing now? What are his heart rate and color?*

"The baby is now apneic. You detect 8 beats in 6 seconds. He is cyanotic."

☐ Slaps foot, flicks heel, or rubs back briefly
☐ *Is the baby breathing now?*

"No, the baby is still apneic."

☐ Chooses correct-sized mask and positions the bag and mask correctly on baby
☐ Checks the seal by ventilating 2 to 3 times at appropriate pressure and observes for chest movement
☐ *Is the chest rising?*

"No, the chest is not rising."
States the need to check each of the following:
☐ Repositions head and reapplies face mask
☐ Checks for and removes secretions
☐ Ventilates with mouth slightly open
☐ Increases ventilation pressure
☐ Considers endotracheal intubation
☐ *Now is the chest rising?*

"Yes, the chest is rising."

☐ Ventilates 30 seconds at a rate of 40-60 times per minute
☐ Achieves visible rise and fall of the chest
☐ Notes need for and inserts orogastric tube if ventilation is required for longer than several minutes   ☐
☐ Counts heart rate by palpating the cord or auscultating the chest for 6 seconds   ☐
     What is the baby's heart rate?

"You detect 5 beats in 6 seconds."

☐ *The baby's heart rate is 50 bpm. I need help to administer chest compressions.*

Learner #1   **Learner #2**

☐ Continues positive-pressure ventilation with 100% oxygen
  Locates appropriate position on lower one-third of baby's sternum   ☐
  Provides firm support for baby's back   ☐
  Uses fingertips of middle and index or ring fingers OR uses distal portion of both thumbs   ☐
  Compresses sternum approximately one-third of the anterior-posterior diameter of the chest   ☐
  Counts cadence of "One-and-Two-and-Three-and-Breathe-and…"   ☐
☐ Ensures that baby is ventilated during the pause after every third compression
  After 30 seconds of chest compressions, checks the heart rate by palpation for 6 seconds while   ☐
    ventilation continues
  What is the baby's heart rate?

"You detect no pulsations."

☐ Stops the ventilations
  Checks heart rate by auscultation for 6 seconds   ☐
  What is the baby's heart rate?

"You detect 5 beats in 6 seconds."

  The baby's heart rate is 50 bpm. We should resume ventilations and chest compressions and make
    sure that we:
  ☐ Are achieving adequate chest movement
  ☐ Are using 100% oxygen
    Are delivering correct depth of chest compressions   ☐
  ☐ Are adequately coordinating ventilations and chest compressions   ☐
  ☐ Have considered endotracheal intubation
  ☐ Have considered epinephrine

☐ Continues chest compressions and ventilations for 30 seconds   ☐
  Palpates umbilical pulse for 6 seconds while positive-pressure ventilation continues   ☐
  What is the baby's heart rate?

"You detect 8 beats in 6 seconds."

  The baby's heart rate is 80 bpm. We can stop chest compressions.   ☐
☐ Continues ventilation for 30 seconds
  Palpates umbilical pulse for 6 seconds while positive-pressure ventilation continues   ☐
  What is the baby's heart rate? Is the baby breathing yet? What is his color?   ☐

"You count 12 beats in 6 seconds. The baby is breathing. His color is dusky."

☐ Gradually discontinues positive-pressure ventilation
☐ Provides tactile stimulation
☐ Gives free-flow oxygen via an oxygen mask, oxygen tubing, or mask of a flow-inflating bag
☐ *Is the baby pink and breathing?*

"Yes, he is pink and breathing."

☐ Withdraws oxygen gradually
☐ Monitors breathing, heart rate, and color
  Is the baby pink in room air?

"Yes, he is pink in room air."

☐ *The baby has been adequately resuscitated, but should be moved to an area where ongoing care*
  and monitoring can be provided.

Performance Checklist
Megacode — Part B

Name _____ Instructor _____ Date _____

This section includes responsibilities for up to three learners: one who ventilates, one who provides chest compressions, and one who administers medications. The location of the check box indicates which learner is responsible for each activity. Each learner may be asked to demonstrate skills in each role.

Instructor's statements are in quotes. Learner's questions and correct responses are in bold type. Instructor should check boxes as the learner answers correctly.

"You are called to attend the birth of a newborn soon to be delivered by emergency cesarean section for severe fetal distress. The mother has suffered abdominal trauma in an automobile accident. She is reportedly leaking blood-tinged amniotic fluid that also contains particles of meconium. The fetus is thought to be close to term. Demonstrate how you would prepare for and resuscitate this newborn."

☐ **Requests extra personnel to be present for delivery**
☐ **Indicates use of standard precautions as appropriate to local regulations**
☐ **Locates and checks function of stethoscope**

Warm
☐ **Turns on radiant warmer**
☐ **Ensures availability of warm linen/towels**

Position; clear airway
☐ **Ensures availability of shoulder roll**
☐ **Assembles laryngoscope and blade size 1 (term)**
☐ **Ensures bright light in laryngoscope**
☐ **Prepares endotracheal tube, size 3.5, and has other sizes available**
☐ **Locates and prepares stylet (optional)**
☐ **Locates meconium aspirator device**
☐ **Locates bulb syringe**
☐ **Ensures function of mechanical suction device with vacuum set at 100 mm Hg**

Oxygenate and Ventilate
☐ **Ensures presence and function of equipment for free-flow oxygen.**
☐ **Ensures that oxygen tubing is attached to flowmeter and bag.**
☐ **Turns on flowmeter to 5 L/min.**
☐ **If self-inflating bag used,**
  • **Ensures that reservoir is attached.**
  • **Checks function of valve assembly and pressure release valve.**
☐ **Checks function of oxygen bag by creating seal with mask against palm of hand. When bag inflates, desired pressure is created.**

☐ **Checks function of pressure manometer on flow-inflating bag (optional on self-inflating bag).**
☐ **If bag is not working properly, obtains and tests another.**
☐ **Locates tape or endotracheal tube securing device.**
☐ **Locates scissors.**

Medicate
☐ **Checks expiration date and concentration of 1:10,000 epinephrine**
☐ **Locates syringes and supplies necessary for desired instillation method of epinephrine**
☐ **Locates and checks expiration dates and concentrations of additional medications**
  • **Normal saline**
  • **Supplies for emergency umbilical venous catheter placement**
  • **4.2% sodium bicarbonate**
☐ **Locates medication labels and waterproof marker**
☐ **Locates code sheet for recording activities**

"The baby's oropharynx is suctioned after delivery of the head, but upon complete delivery she is limp and unresponsive. She is then handed to you. Demonstrate and explain what you would do. You may ask me about specific details of the baby's condition."

Learner #1   **Learner #2**

☐ *Is meconium present? What is the baby's breathing, tone, and heart rate?*

"Yes, there is meconium on the skin. The baby is limp, apneic and has a heart rate of 90."

 The baby is meconium stained and is not vigorous; she requires tracheal suction.

☐ **Correctly positions manikin on radiant warmer**   ☐
☐ **Provides/uses free-flow oxygen**   ☐
 Provides suction when requested   ☐
☐ **Inserts blade into mouth, holding laryngoscope correctly**
 Applies laryngeal pressure correctly if asked   ☐
☐ **Inserts tube into trachea**
☐ **Removes laryngoscope (and stylet if used)**
☐ **Connects (or assists with) meconium aspirator**   ☐
☐ **Withdraws tube while applying suction**
☐ **Performs entire procedure within 20 seconds**

 Now I will proceed with the initial steps.

☐ **Dries body and head**
☐ **Removes wet linen**
☐ **Stimulates and repositions baby with neck slightly extended**
☐ **Administers oxygen as necessary**

 Counts heart rate by palpating the cord or auscultating the chest for 6 seconds   ☐
☐ *Is the baby breathing now? What are his heart rate and color?*

"The baby is apneic. You detect 7 beats in 6 seconds. She is cyanotic."

☐ **Slaps foot, flicks heel, or rubs back briefly**
☐ *Is the baby breathing now?*

"No, the baby is still apneic."

☐ **Chooses correct-sized mask and positions the bag and mask correctly on baby**
☐ **Checks the seal by ventilating 2 to 3 times at appropriate pressure and observes for chest movement**
 Is the chest rising?

"No, the chest is not rising."
 States the need to check each of the following:
☐ **Repositions head and reapplies face mask**
☐ **Checks for and removes secretions**
☐ **Ventilates with mouth slightly open**
☐ **Increases ventilation pressure**
☐ **Considers endotracheal intubation**
☐ *Now is the chest rising?*

"Yes, the chest is rising."

☐ Ventilates 30 seconds at a rate of 40 to 60 times per minute
☐ Achieves visible rise and fall of the chest
☐ Notes need for and inserts orogastric tube if ventilation is required for longer than several minutes ☐
   Counts heart rate by palpating the cord or auscultating the chest for 6 seconds ☐
   What is the baby's heart rate?

"You detect 5 beats in 6 seconds."

☐ *The heart rate is 50 bpm. This baby needs chest compressions. My assistant will begin chest compressions while I continue to ventilate.*

   Locates appropriate position on lower one-third of baby's sternum ☐
   Provides firm support for baby's back ☐
   Uses fingertips of middle and index or ring fingers OR uses distal portion of both thumbs ☐
   Compresses sternum approximately one-third of the anterior-posterior diameter of the chest ☐
   Counts cadence of "One-and-Two-and-Three-and-Breathe-and…" ☐
☐ Ensures that baby is ventilated during the pause after every third compression
   After 30 seconds of chest compressions, checks the heart rate by palpation for 6 seconds
      while ventilation continues ☐
   What is the baby's heart rate?

"You detect no pulsations."

☐ Stops the ventilations
   Checks heart rate by auscultation for 6 seconds ☐
   What is the baby's heart rate?

"You detect 5 beats in 6 seconds."

   The baby's heart rate is 50 bpm. We should resume ventilation and chest compressions and make sure that we:
☐ Are achieving adequate chest movement
☐ Are using 100% oxygen
   Are delivering correct depth of chest compressions ☐
☐ Are adequately coordinating ventilation and chest compressions ☐
☐ If all are correct, have considered endotracheal intubation
☐ Have considered epinephrine administration

   Chest compressions cease during intubation ☐
☐ Provides/uses free-flow oxygen ☐
   Provides suction when requested ☐
☐ Inserts blade into mouth, holding laryngoscope correctly
   Applies laryngeal pressure correctly if asked ☐
☐ Inserts tube into trachea
☐ Removes laryngoscope (and stylet if used) while firmly holding the tube in place at the correct "tip-to-lip" measurement
☐ Attaches endotracheal tube to bag and inflates lungs ☐
☐ Completes procedure in 20 seconds OR
☐ Resumes chest compressions and bag-and-mask ventilation, then repeats attempt ☐
☐ Correctly states steps for confirming placement (chest rise, bilateral breath sounds, mist inside tube, no increasing gastric distention) and considers use of CO_2 detector

Learner #1	Learner #2	Learner #3

☐ Checks the heart rate by palpating the umbilical cord for 6 seconds (ventilations continue) or auscultates the chest if no pulsations are detected (ventilations cease)
What is the baby's heart rate?

"You detect 5 beats in 6 seconds."

☐ *The baby's heart rate is 50 bpm. We will resume chest compressions and ventilation and another assistant will administer epinephrine down the endotracheal tube. What is this baby's estimated weight?*

"The baby appears to be approximately 3.0 Kg."

☐ *The dosage range for 1:10,000 epinephrine for this 3.0 kg infant is 0.3 to 0.9 mL. We will draw up (.3 to .9) mL in the syringe.*

☐ Demonstrates how to draw up epinephrine in the syringe and attaches label
☐ Demonstrates administration of epinephrine via endotracheal tube
Directly into the endotracheal tube OR
Via a 5F feeding tube or catheter inserted down the endotracheal tube
☐ Reattaches bag to endotracheal tube and resumes positive-pressure ventilation ☐ and chest compressions for 30 seconds
☐ Checks the heart rate by palpating the umbilical cord for 6 seconds ☐ (ventilations continue) or auscultating the chest if no pulsations are detected (ventilations cease)
What is the heart rate?

"You detect 7 beats in 6 seconds."

☐ *The baby's heart rate is 70 bpm. We can stop chest compressions and* ☐ *continue ventilation.*
☐ Continues ventilation at rate of 40 to 60 breaths per minute for 30 seconds

☐ Checks the heart rate by palpating the umbilical cord for 6 seconds ☐ (ventilations continue) or auscultating the chest if no pulsations are detected (ventilations cease)
What is the baby's heart rate? Is she breathing on her own? What is her color?

"You detect 12 beats in 6 seconds. The baby is taking an occasional breath on her own. Her color has improved, though she is still pale. She remains limp."

☐ *I will continue positive-pressure ventilation. We will secure the endotracheal tube now that things are under control.*
☐ States centimeter marking at level of upper lip
☐ Secures tube while maintaining proper position

☐ *The baby has been adequately resuscitated, but should be moved to an area where ongoing care and monitoring can be provided.*

Overall

☐ Communicated and performed well as a team ☐ ☐
Recorded all activities ☐

Appendix

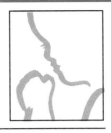

International Guidelines for Neonatal Resuscitation: An Excerpt From the Guidelines 2000 for Cardiopulmonary Resuscitation and Emergency Cardiovascular Care: International Consensus on Science

ABSTRACT. The International Guidelines 2000 Conference on Cardiopulmonary Resuscitation (CPR) and Emergency Cardiac Care (ECC) formulated new evidenced-based recommendations for neonatal resuscitation. These guidelines comprehensively update the last recommendations, published in 1992 after the Fifth National Conference on CPR and ECC.

As a result of the evidence evaluation process, significant changes occurred in the recommended management routines for:

• Meconium-stained amniotic fluid: If the newly born infant has absent or depressed respirations, heart rate <100 beats per minute (bpm), or poor muscle tone, direct tracheal suctioning should be performed to remove meconium from the airway.

• Preventing heat loss: Hyperthermia should be avoided.

• Oxygenation and ventilation: 100% oxygen is recommended for assisted ventilation; however, if supplemental oxygen is unavailable, positive-pressure ventilation should be initiated with room air. The laryngeal mask airway may serve as an effective alternative for establishing an airway if bag-mask ventilation is ineffective or attempts at intubation have failed. Exhaled CO_2 detection can be useful in the secondary confirmation of endotracheal intubation.

• Chest compressions: Compressions should be administered if the heart rate is absent or remains <60 bpm despite adequate assisted ventilation for 30 seconds. The 2-thumb, encircling-hands method of chest compression is preferred, with a depth of compression one third the anterior-posterior diameter of the chest and sufficient to generate a palpable pulse.

• Medications, volume expansion, and vascular access: Epinephrine in a dose of 0.01–0.03 mg/kg (0.1–0.3 mL/kg of 1:10,000 solution) should be administered if the heart rate remains <60 bpm after a minimum of 30 seconds of adequate ventilation and chest compressions. Emergency volume expansion may be accomplished with an isotonic crystalloid solution or O-negative red blood cells; albumin-containing solutions are no longer the fluid of choice for initial volume expansion. Intraosseous access can serve as an alternative route for medications/volume expansion if umbilical or other direct venous access is not readily available.

• Noninitiation and discontinuation of resuscitation: There are circumstances (relating to gestational age, birth weight, known underlying condition, lack of response to interventions) in which noninitiation or discontinuation of resuscitation in the delivery room may be appropriate. *Pediatrics* 2000;106(3). URL: http://www.pediatrics.org/cgi/content/full/106/3/e29; *neonatal resuscitation.*

INTRODUCTORY FRAMEWORK FOR NEONATAL RESUSCITATION GUIDELINES

The Neonatal Resuscitation Guidelines present the recommendations of the International Guidelines 2000 Conference on Cardiopulmonary Resuscitation (CPR) and Emergency Cardiovascular Care (ECC). The Guidelines 2000 Conference assembled international experts from many fields, including neonatal resuscitation, to comprehensively update existing guidelines through a process of evidence evaluation.

The Neonatal Resuscitation Program Steering Committee (American Academy of Pediatrics), the Pediatric Working Group of the International Liaison Committee on Resuscitation (ILCOR), and the Pediatric Resuscitation Subcommittee of the Emergency Cardiovascular Care Committee (American Heart Association) worked together for 2 years in a systematic process of evidence evaluation and formulation of new recommendations. In 1999 the Pediatric Working Group of ILCOR developed a consensus advisory statement, "Resuscitation of the newly born infant" (*Pediatrics* 1999;103(4). http://www.pediatrics.org/cgi/content/full/103/4/e56). Using questions and controversies identified during the consensus process, members of the participating organizations worked with additional topic experts from various countries to assemble the most current scientific information relating to neonatal resuscitation. A standard worksheet template served as a framework for uniform evaluation of each selected topic. Articles published in peer-reviewed journals were assembled and analyzed individually for relevance to the proposed guideline change and the quality of the evidence presented. Strength of evidence was classified on the basis of the level of evidence, or study design (ie, randomized, controlled trials, prospective observational studies, retrospective observational studies, case series, animal studies, extrapolations, and common sense) and the quality of the methodology (population, techniques, bias, confounders, etc). Integration of evidence at many different levels and of different quality occurred through consensus discussions among experts and formal panel presentation and debate at the Evidence Evaluation Conference (American Heart Association, September 1999). From the integration process emerged a class of recommendation for each proposed guideline, based on the level of evidence and critical assessment of the quality of the studies, as well as the number of studies, consistency of conclusions, outcomes measured, and magnitude of benefit. The proposed guideline

The Neonatal Resuscitation Guidelines, as presented here, constitute only one part of the International Guidelines 2000 for CPR and ECC. Full content of the guidelines, including recommendations for adult, pediatric, and neonatal age groups at both basic and advanced life support levels, appears in a supplement to *Circulation* (2000;102(suppl I):I-343–I-357).

TABLE I. Clinical Interpretation of Classes of Recommendations

Class of Recommendation	Interpretation
Class I	Always acceptable, proven safe, definitely useful
Class IIa	Acceptable, safe, useful (standard of care or intervention of choice)
Class IIb	Acceptable, safe, useful (within the standard of care or an optional or alternative intervention)
Class indeterminate	Preliminary research stage with promising results but insufficient available evidence to support a final class decision
Class III	Unacceptable, no documented benefit, may be harmful

changes, as well as their class of recommendation and level of evidence were presented for final debate and ratification at the Guidelines 2000 Conference (February 2000).

For each new or revised guideline, the class of recommendation, as well as the highest level of evidence (LOE) supporting the recommendation, appears in the text. Table I provides a guide to the clinical interpretation of each class of recommendation. Previous guideline recommendations not originally formulated through evidence-based review remain in place unless there existed a lack of evidence to confirm effectiveness, new evidence to suggest harm or ineffectiveness, or evidence that superior approaches had become available. Although the International Guidelines 2000 present the consensus of experts in the field of resuscitation, use of the guidelines is not mandated or imposed upon an individual or organization. The guidelines represent the most effective practices for resuscitation of the newly born infant, based upon current research, knowledge, and experience. As such they are intended to serve as the foundation for educational programs and national, regional, and local processes which establish standards of practice.

MAJOR GUIDELINES CHANGES

The Pediatric Working Group of the International Liaison Committee on Resuscitation (ILCOR) developed an advisory statement published in 1999. This statement listed the following principles of resuscitation of the newly born:

- Personnel capable of initiating resuscitation should attend every delivery. A minority (fewer than 10%) of newly born infants require active resuscitative interventions to establish a vigorous cry or regular respirations, maintain a heart rate >100 beats per minute (bpm), and achieve good color and tone.
- When meconium is observed in the amniotic fluid, deliver the head, and suction meconium from the hypopharynx on delivery of the head. If the newly born infant has absent or depressed respirations, heart rate <100 bpm, or poor muscle tone, carry out direct tracheal suctioning to remove meconium from the airway.
- Establishment of adequate ventilation should be of primary concern. Provide assisted ventilation with

attention to oxygen delivery, inspiratory time, and effectiveness as judged by chest rise if stimulation does not achieve prompt onset of spontaneous respirations or the heart rate is <100 bpm.
- Provide chest compressions if the heart rate is absent or remains <60 bpm despite adequate assisted ventilation for 30 seconds. Coordinate chest compressions with ventilations at a ratio of 3:1 and a rate of 120 events per minute to achieve approximately 90 compressions and 30 breaths per minute.
- Administer epinephrine if the heart rate remains <60 bpm despite 30 seconds of effective assisted ventilation and circulation (chest compressions).

At the Guidelines 2000 Conference, we made the following recommendations:

Temperature
- Cerebral hypothermia; avoidance of perinatal hyperthermia
  —Avoid hyperthermia (Class III).
  —Although several recent animal and human studies have suggested that selective cerebral hypothermia may protect against brain injury in the asphyxiated infant, we cannot recommend routine implementation of this therapy until appropriate controlled human studies have been performed (Class Indeterminate).

Oxygenation and Ventilation
- Room air versus 100% oxygen during positive-pressure ventilation
  —100% oxygen has been used traditionally for rapid reversal of hypoxia. Although biochemical and preliminary clinical evidence suggests that lower inspired oxygen concentrations may be useful in some settings, data is insufficient to justify a change from the recommendation that 100% oxygen be used if assisted ventilation is required.
  —If supplemental oxygen is unavailable and positive-pressure ventilation is required, use room air (Class Indeterminate).
- Laryngeal mask as an alternative method of establishing an airway
  —When used by appropriately trained providers, the laryngeal mask airway may be an effective alternative for establishing an airway during resuscitation of the newly born infant, particularly if bag-mask ventilation is ineffective or attempts at tracheal intubation have failed (Class Indeterminate).
- Confirmation of tracheal tube placement by exhaled CO_2 detection
  —Exhaled CO_2 detection can be useful in the secondary confirmation of tracheal intubation in the newly born, particularly when clinical assessment is equivocal (Class Indeterminate).

Chest Compressions
- Preferred technique for chest compressions
  —Two thumb–encircling hands chest compression is the preferred technique for chest com-

pressions in newly born infants and older infants when size permits (Class IIb).
—For chest compressions, we recommend a relative depth of compression (one third of the anterior-posterior diameter of the chest) rather than an absolute depth. Chest compressions should be sufficiently deep to generate a palpable pulse.

Medications, Volume Expansion, and Vascular Access
- Epinephrine dose
  —Administer epinephrine if the heart rate remains <60 bpm after a minimum of 30 seconds of adequate ventilation and chest compressions (Class I).
  —Epinephrine administration is particularly indicated in the presence of asystole.
- Choice of fluid for acute volume expansion
  —Emergency volume expansion may be accomplished by an isotonic crystalloid solution such as normal saline or Ringer's lactate. O-negative red blood cells may be used if the need for blood replacement is anticipated before birth (Class IIb).
  —Albumin-containing solutions are no longer the fluid of choice for initial volume expansion because their availability is limited, they introduce a risk of infectious disease, and an association with increased mortality has been observed.
- Alternative routes for vascular access
  —Intraosseous access can be used as an alternative route for medications/volume expansion if umbilical or other direct venous access is not readily available (Class IIb).

Ethics
- Noninitiation and discontinuation of resuscitation
  —There are circumstances (relating to gestational age, birth weight, known underlying condition, lack of response to interventions) in which noninitiation or discontinuation of resuscitation in the delivery room may be appropriate (Class IIb).

INTRODUCTION

Resuscitation of the newly born infant presents a different set of challenges than resuscitation of the adult or even the older infant or child. The transition from placental gas exchange in a liquid-filled intrauterine environment to spontaneous breathing of air requires dramatic physiological changes in the infant within the first minutes to hours after birth.

Approximately 5% to 10% of the newly born population require some degree of active resuscitation at birth (eg, stimulation to breathe),[1] and approximately 1% to 10% born in the hospital are reported to require assisted ventilation.[2] More than 5 million neonatal deaths occur worldwide each year. It has been estimated that birth asphyxia accounts for 19% of these deaths, suggesting that the outcome might be improved for more than 1 million infants per year through implementation of simple resuscitative techniques.[3] Although the need for resuscitation of the newly born infant often can be predicted, such cir-

cumstances may arise suddenly and may occur in facilities that do not routinely provide neonatal intensive care. Thus, it is essential that the knowledge and skills required for resuscitation be taught to all providers of neonatal care.

With adequate anticipation, it is possible to optimize the delivery setting with appropriately prepared equipment and trained personnel who are capable of functioning as a team during neonatal resuscitation. At least 1 person skilled in initiating neonatal resuscitation should be present at every delivery. An additional skilled person capable of performing a complete resuscitation should be immediately available.

Neonatal resuscitation can be divided into 4 categories of action:

- Basic steps, including rapid assessment and initial steps in stabilization
- Ventilation, including bag-mask or bag-tube ventilation
- Chest compressions
- Administration of medications or fluids

Tracheal intubation may be required during any of these steps. All newly born infants require rapid assessment, including examination for the presence of meconium in the amniotic fluid or on the skin; evaluation of breathing, muscle tone, and color; and classification of gestational age as term or preterm. Newly born infants with a normal rapid assessment require only routine care (warmth, clearing the airway, drying). All others receive the initial steps, including warmth, clearing the airway, drying, positioning, stimulation to initiate or improve respirations, and oxygen as necessary.

Subsequent evaluation and intervention are based on a triad of characteristics: (1) respirations, (2) heart rate, and (3) color. Most newly born infants require only the basic steps, but for those who require further intervention, the most crucial action is establishment of adequate ventilation. Only a very small percentage will need chest compressions and medications.[4]

Certain special circumstances have unique implications for resuscitation of the newly born infant. Care of the infant after resuscitation includes not only supportive care but also ongoing monitoring and appropriate diagnostic evaluation. In certain clinical circumstances, noninitiation or discontinuation of resuscitation in the delivery room may be appropriate. Finally, it is important to document resuscitation interventions and responses in order to understand an individual infant's pathophysiology as well as to improve resuscitation performance and study resuscitation outcomes.[5–8]

BACKGROUND

Changes in Neonatal Resuscitation Guidelines, 1992 to 2000

The ILCOR Pediatric Working Group consists of representatives from the American Heart Association (AHA), European Resuscitation Council (ERC), Heart and Stroke Foundation of Canada (HSFC),

Australian Resuscitation Council (ARC), New Zealand Resuscitation Council (NZRC), Resuscitation Council of Southern Africa (RCSA), and Council of Latin America for Resuscitation (CLAR). Members of the Neonatal Resuscitation Program (NRP) Steering Committee of the American Academy of Pediatrics (AAP) and representatives of the World Health Organization (WHO) joined the ILCOR Pediatric Working Group to extend existing advisory recommendations for pediatric and neonatal basic life support[9] to comprehensive basic and advanced resuscitation for the newly born.[10] Careful review of the guidelines of constituent organizations[11–17] and current international literature formed the basis for the 1999 ILCOR advisory statement.[10] We have included consensus recommendations from that statement at the beginning of this document.

Using questions and controversies identified during the ILCOR process, the Neonatal Resuscitation Program Steering Committee (AAP), the Pediatric Working Group (ILCOR), and the Pediatric Resuscitation Subcommittee of the Emergency Cardiovascular Care Committee (AHA) carried out further evidence evaluation. At the Evidence Evaluation Conference and International Guidelines 2000 Conference on CPR and ECC, these groups and panels of international experts and participants developed additional recommendations. The International Guidelines 2000 recommendations form the basis of this document.

Definition of "Newly Born," "Neonate," and "Infant"

Although the guidelines for neonatal resuscitation focus on newly born infants, most of the principles are applicable throughout the neonatal period and early infancy. The term "newly born" refers specifically to the infant in *the first minutes to hours after birth*. The term "neonate" is generally defined as an infant during the first 28 days of life. Infancy includes the neonatal period and extends through 12 months of age.

Unique Physiology of the Newly Born

The transition from fetal to extrauterine life is characterized by a series of unique physiological events: the lungs change from fluid-filled to air-filled, pulmonary blood flow increases dramatically, and intracardiac and extracardiac shunts (foramen ovale and ductus arteriosus) initially reverse direction and subsequently close. Such physiological considerations affect resuscitative interventions in the newly born.

For initial lung expansion, fluid-filled alveoli may require higher ventilation pressures than are commonly used in rescue breathing during infancy.[18,19] Physical expansion of the lungs, with establishment of functional residual capacity and increase in alveolar oxygen tension, both mediate the critical decrease in pulmonary vascular resistance and result in an increase in pulmonary blood flow after birth. Failure to normalize pulmonary vascular resistance may result in persistence of right-to-left intracardiac and extracardiac shunts (persistent pulmonary hypertension). Failure to adequately expand alveolar spaces may result in intrapulmonary shunting of blood with resultant hypoxemia. In addition to disordered cardiopulmonary transition, disruption of the fetoplacental circulation also may render the newly born at risk for resuscitation because of acute blood loss.

Developmental considerations at various gestational ages also influence pulmonary pathology and resuscitation physiology in the newly born. Surfactant deficiency in the premature infant alters lung compliance and resistance.[20] Meconium passed into the amniotic fluid may be aspirated, leading to airway obstruction. Complications of meconium aspiration are particularly likely in infants small for gestational age and those born post term or with significant perinatal compromise.[21]

Although certain physiological features are unique to the newly born, others pertain to infants throughout the neonatal period and into the first months of life. Severe illness due to a wide variety of conditions continues to manifest as disturbances in respiratory function (cyanosis, apnea, respiratory failure). Convalescing preterm infants with chronic lung disease often require significant ventilatory support regardless of the etiology of their need for resuscitation. Persistent pulmonary hypertension, persistent patency of the ductus arteriosus, and intracardiac shunts may produce symptoms during the neonatal period or even into infancy. Thus, many of the considerations and interventions that apply to the newly born may remain important for days, weeks, or months after birth.

The point at which neonatal resuscitation guidelines should be replaced by pediatric resuscitation protocols varies for individual patients. Objective data is lacking on optimal compression-ventilation ratios by age and disease state. However, infants with acute or chronic lung disease may benefit from a lower compression-ventilation ratio well into infancy. For these infants, continued use of some aspects of the neonatal guidelines is reasonable. Conversely, a neonate with a cardiac arrhythmia resulting in poor perfusion requires use of protocols more fully detailed in pediatric advanced life support. Factors of age, pathophysiology, and caregiver training should be evaluated for each patient and the most appropriate resuscitation routines and care setting identified.

ANTICIPATION OF RESUSCITATION NEED

Anticipation, adequate preparation, accurate evaluation, and prompt initiation of support are the critical steps to successful neonatal resuscitation.

Communication

Appropriate preparation for an anticipated high-risk delivery requires communication between the person(s) caring for the mother and those responsible for resuscitation of the newly born. Communication among caregivers should include details of antepartum and intrapartum maternal medical conditions and treatment as well as specific indicators of fetal condition (fetal heart rate monitoring, lung maturity, ultrasonography). Table 1 lists examples of the

TABLE 1. Conditions Associated With Risk to Newborns

Antepartum risk factors
Maternal diabetes
Pregnancy-induced hypertension
Chronic hypertension
Chronic maternal illness
  Cardiovascular
  Thyroid
  Neurological
  Pulmonary
  Renal
Anemia or isoimmunization
Previous fetal or neonatal death
Bleeding in second or third trimester
Maternal infection
Polyhydramnios
Oligohydramnios
Premature rupture of membranes
Post-term gestation
Multiple gestation
Size-dates discrepancy
Drug therapy, eg,
  Lithium carbonate
  Magnesium
  Adrenergic-blocking drugs
Maternal substance abuse
Fetal malformation
Diminished fetal activity
No prenatal care
Age <16 or >35 years

Intrapartum risk factors
Emergency cesarean section
Forceps or vacuum-assisted delivery
Breech or other abnormal presentation
Premature labor
Precipitous labor
Chorioamnionitis
Prolonged rupture of membranes (>18 hours before delivery)
Prolonged labor (>24 hours)
Prolonged second stage of labor (>2 hours)
Fetal bradycardia
Non-reassuring fetal heart rate patterns
Use of general anesthesia
Uterine tetany
Narcotics administered to mother within 4 hours of delivery
Meconium-stained amniotic fluid
Prolapsed cord
Abruptio placentae
Placenta previa

---

antepartum and intrapartum circumstances that place the newly born infant at risk.

PREPARATION FOR DELIVERY

Personnel

Personnel capable of initiating resuscitation should attend every delivery. At least 1 such person should be responsible solely for care of the infant. A person capable of carrying out a complete resuscitation should be immediately available for normal low-risk deliveries and in attendance for all deliveries considered high risk. More than 1 experienced person should attend an anticipated high-risk delivery. Resuscitation of a severely depressed newly born infant requires at least 2 persons, 1 to ventilate and intubate if necessary and another to monitor heart rate and perform chest compressions if required. A team of 3 or more persons with designated roles is highly desirable during an extensive resuscitation including medication administration. A separate team should be present for each infant of a multiple gestation. Each resuscitation team should have an identified leader, and all team members should have specifically defined roles.

Equipment

Although the need for resuscitation at birth often can be predicted by risk factors, for many infants resuscitation cannot be anticipated.[22] Therefore, a clean and warm environment with a complete inventory of resuscitation equipment and drugs should be maintained at hand and in fully operational condition wherever deliveries occur. Table 2 presents a list of suggested neonatal supplies, medications, and equipment.

Standard precautions should be followed carefully in delivery areas, where exposure to blood and body fluids is likely. All fluids from patients should be treated as potentially infectious. Personnel should wear gloves and other appropriate protective barriers when handling newly born infants or contaminated equipment. Techniques involving mouth suction by the healthcare provider should not be used.

EVALUATION

Determination of the need for resuscitative efforts should begin immediately after birth and proceed throughout the resuscitation process. An initial complex of signs (meconium in the amniotic fluid or on the skin, cry or respirations, muscle tone, color, term or preterm gestation) should be evaluated rapidly and simultaneously by visual inspection. Actions are dictated by integrated evaluation rather than by evaluation of a single vital sign, followed by action on the result, and then evaluation of the next sign (sequential action). Evaluation and intervention for the newly born are often simultaneous processes, especially when >1 trained provider is present. To enhance educational retention, this process is often taught as a sequence of distinct steps. The appropriate response to abnormal findings also depends on the time elapsed since birth and how the infant has responded to previous resuscitative interventions.

Response to Extrauterine Environment

Most newly born infants will respond to the stimulation of the extrauterine environment with strong inspiratory efforts, a vigorous cry, and movement of all extremities. If these responses are intact, color improves steadily from cyanotic or dusky to pink, and heart rate can be assumed to be adequate. The infant who responds vigorously to the extrauterine environment and who is term can remain with the mother to receive routine care (warmth, clearing the airway, drying). Indications for further assessment under a radiant warmer and possible intervention include

- Meconium in the amniotic fluid or on the skin
- Absent or weak responses
- Persistent cyanosis
- Preterm birth

Further assessment of the newly born infant is based on the triad of respiration, heart rate, and color.

TABLE 2. Neonatal Resuscitation Supplies and Equipment

Suction equipment
  Bulb syringe
  Mechanical suction and tubing
  Suction catheters, 5F or 6F, 8F, and 10F or 12F
  8F feeding tube and 20-mL syringe
  Meconium aspiration device
Bag-and-mask equipment
  Neonatal resuscitation bag with a pressure-release valve or pressure manometer (the bag must
    be capable of delivering 90% to 100% oxygen)
  Face masks, newborn and premature sizes (masks with cushioned rim preferred)
  Oxygen with flowmeter (flow rate up to 10 L/min) and tubing (including portable oxygen
    cylinders)
Intubation equipment
  Laryngoscope with straight blades, No. 0 (preterm) and No. 1 (term)
  Extra bulbs and batteries for laryngoscope
  Tracheal tubes, 2.5, 3.0, 3.5, and 4.0 mm ID
  Stylet (optional)
  Scissors
  Tape or securing device for tracheal tube
  Alcohol sponges
  CO_2 detector (optional)
  Laryngeal mask airway (optional)
Medications
  Epinephrine 1:10 000 (0.1 mg/mL)—3-mL or 10-mL ampules
  Isotonic crystalloid (normal saline or Ringer's lactate) for volume expansion—100 or 250 mL
  Sodium bicarbonate 4.2% (5 mEq/10 mL)—10-mL ampules
  Naloxone hydrochloride 0.4 mg/mL—1-mL ampules; or 1.0 mg/mL—2-mL ampules
  Normal saline, 30 mL
  Dextrose 10%, 250 mL
  Normal saline "fish" or "bullet" (optional)
  Feeding tube, 5F (optional)
  Umbilical vessel catheterization supplies
    Sterile gloves
    Scalpel or scissors
    Povidone-iodine solution
    Umbilical tape
    Umbilical catheters, 3.5F, 5F
    Three-way stopcock
  Syringes, 1, 3, 5, 10, 20, and 50 mL
  Needles, 25-, 21-, and 18-gauge or puncture device for needleless system
Miscellaneous
  Gloves and appropriate personal protection
  Radiant warmer or other heat source
  Firm, padded resuscitation surface
  Clock (timer optional)
  Warmed linens
  Stethoscope
  Tape, ½ or ¾ inch
  Cardiac monitor and electrodes and/or pulse oximeter with probe (optional for delivery room)
  Oropharyngeal airways

Respiration

After initial respiratory efforts, the newly born infant should be able to establish regular respirations sufficient to improve color and maintain a heart rate >100 bpm. Gasping and apnea are signs that indicate the need for assisted ventilation.[23]

Heart Rate

Heart rate is determined by listening to the precordium with a stethoscope or feeling pulsations at the base of the umbilical cord. Central and peripheral pulses in the neck and extremities are often difficult to feel in infants,[24,25] but the umbilical pulse is readily accessible in the newly born and permits assessment of heart rate without interruption of ventilation for auscultation. If pulsations cannot be felt at the base of the cord, auscultation of the precordium should be performed. Heart rate should be consistently >100 bpm in an uncompromised newly born infant. An increasing

or decreasing heart rate also can provide evidence of improvement or deterioration.

Color

An uncompromised newly born infant will be able to maintain a pink color of the mucous membranes without supplemental oxygen. Central cyanosis is determined by examining the face, trunk, and mucous membranes. Acrocyanosis is usually a normal finding at birth and is not a reliable indicator of hypoxemia, but it may indicate other conditions, such as cold stress. Pallor may be a sign of decreased cardiac output, severe anemia, hypovolemia, hypothermia, or acidosis.

TECHNIQUES OF RESUSCITATION

The techniques of neonatal resuscitation are discussed below and are outlined in the algorithm (see Figure).

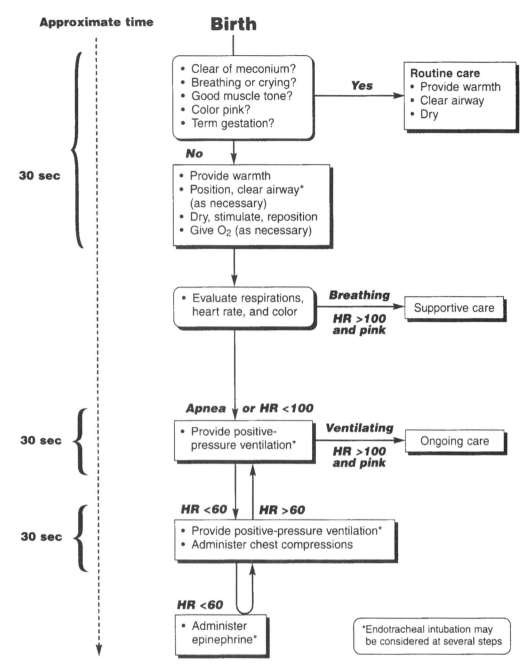

Approximate time

Birth

- Clear of meconium?
- Breathing or crying?
- Good muscle tone?
- Color pink?
- Term gestation?

Yes →

Routine care
- Provide warmth
- Clear airway
- Dry

No

30 sec

- Provide warmth
- Position, clear airway* (as necessary)
- Dry, stimulate, reposition
- Give O$_2$ (as necessary)

- Evaluate respirations, heart rate, and color

Breathing
HR >100 and pink → Supportive care

Apnea or *HR <100*

30 sec

- Provide positive-pressure ventilation*

Ventilating
HR >100 and pink → Ongoing care

HR <60   *HR >60*

30 sec

- Provide positive-pressure ventilation*
- Administer chest compressions

HR <60

- Administer epinephrine*

*Endotracheal intubation may be considered at several steps

Algorithm for resuscitation of the newly born infant.

Basic Steps

Warmth

Preventing heat loss in the newly born is vital because cold stress can increase oxygen consumption and impede effective resuscitation.[26,27] Hyperthermia should be avoided, however, because it is associated with perinatal respiratory depression[28,29] (Class III, level of evidence [LOE] 3). Whenever possible, deliver the infant in a warm, draft-free area. Placing the infant under a radiant warmer, rapidly drying the skin, removing wet linen immediately, and wrapping the infant in prewarmed blankets will reduce heat loss. Another strategy for reducing heat loss is placing the dried infant skin-to-skin on the mother's chest or abdomen to use her body as a heat source.

Recent animal and human studies have suggested that selective (cerebral) hypothermia of the asphyxiated infant may protect against brain injury.[30–32] Although this is a promising area of research, we cannot recommend routine implementation until appropriate controlled studies in humans have been performed (Class Indeterminate, LOE 2).

Clearing the Airway

The infant's airway is cleared by positioning of the infant and removal of secretions if needed.

Positioning

The newly born infant should be placed supine or lying on its side, with the head in a neutral or slightly extended position. If respiratory efforts are present but not producing effective tidal ventilation, often the airway is obstructed; immediate efforts must be made to correct overextension or flexion or to remove secretions. A blanket or towel placed under the shoulders may be helpful in maintaining proper head position.

Suctioning

If time permits, the person assisting delivery of the infant should suction the infant's nose and mouth with a bulb syringe after delivery of the shoulders but before delivery of the chest. Healthy, vigorous, newly born infants generally do not require suctioning after delivery.[33] Secretions may be wiped from the nose and mouth with gauze or a towel. If suctioning is necessary, clear secretions first from the mouth and then the nose with a bulb syringe or suction catheter (8F or 10F). Aggressive pharyngeal suction can cause laryngeal spasm and vagal bradycardia[34] and delay the onset of spontaneous breathing. In the absence of meconium or blood, limit mechanical suction with a catheter in depth and duration. Negative pressure of the suction apparatus should not exceed 100 mm Hg (13.3 kPa or 136 cm H_2O). If copious secretions are present, the infant's head may be turned to the side, and suctioning may help clear the airway.

Clearing the Airway of Meconium

Approximately 12% of deliveries are complicated by the presence of meconium in the amniotic fluid.[35] When the amniotic fluid is meconium-stained, suction the mouth, pharynx, and nose as soon as the head is delivered (intrapartum suctioning) regardless of whether the meconium is thin or thick.[36] Either a large-bore suction catheter (12F to 14F) or bulb syringe can be used.[37] Thorough suctioning of the nose, mouth, and posterior pharynx before delivery of the body appears to decrease the risk of meconium-aspiration syndrome.[36] Nevertheless, a significant number (20% to 30%) of meconium-stained infants will have meconium in the trachea despite such suctioning and in the absence of spontaneous respirations.[38,39] This suggests the occurrence of in utero aspiration and the need for tracheal suctioning after delivery in *depressed* infants.

If the fluid contains meconium and the infant has absent or depressed respirations, decreased muscle tone, or heart rate <100 bpm, perform direct laryngoscopy immediately after birth for suctioning of residual meconium from the hypopharynx (under direct vision) and intubation/suction of the trachea.[40,41] There is evidence that tracheal suctioning of the vigorous infant with meconium-stained fluid does not improve outcome and may cause complications (Class I, LOE 1).[42,43] Warmth can be provided by a radiant heater; however, drying and stimulation generally should be delayed in such infants. Accomplish tracheal suctioning by applying suction directly to a tracheal tube as it is withdrawn from the airway. Repeat intubation and suctioning until little additional meconium is recovered or until the heart rate indicates that resuscitation must proceed without delay. If the infant's heart rate or respiration is severely depressed, it may be necessary to institute positive-pressure ventilation despite the presence of some meconium in the airway. Suction catheters inserted through the tracheal tube may be too small to accomplish initial removal of particulate meconium; subsequent use of suction catheters inserted through a tracheal tube may be adequate to continue removal of meconium. Delay gastric suctioning to prevent aspiration of swallowed meconium until initial resuscitation is complete. Meconium-stained infants who develop apnea or respiratory distress should receive tracheal suctioning before positive-pressure ventilation, even if they are initially vigorous.

Tactile Stimulation

Drying and suctioning produce enough stimulation to initiate effective respirations in most newly born infants. If an infant fails to establish spontaneous and effective respirations after drying with a towel or gentle rubbing of the back, flicking the soles of the feet may initiate spontaneous respirations. Avoid more vigorous methods of stimulation. Tactile stimulation may initiate spontaneous respirations in newly born infants who are experiencing primary apnea. If these efforts do not result in prompt onset of effective ventilation, discontinue them because the infant is in secondary apnea and positive-pressure ventilation will be required.[23]

Oxygen Administration

Hypoxia is nearly always present in a newly born infant who requires resuscitation. Therefore, if cyanosis, bradycardia, or other signs of distress are noted in a breathing newborn during stabilization, administration of 100% oxygen is indicated while determining the need for additional intervention. Free-flow oxygen can be delivered through a face mask and flow-inflating bag, an oxygen mask, or a hand cupped around oxygen tubing. The oxygen source should deliver at least 5 L/min, and the oxygen should be held close to the face to maximize the inhaled concentration. Many self-inflating bags will not passively deliver sufficient oxygen flow (ie, when not being squeezed). The goal of supplemental oxygen use should be normoxia; sufficient oxygen should be administered to achieve pink color in the mucous membranes. If cyanosis returns when supplemental oxygen is withdrawn, post-resuscitation care should include monitoring of administered oxygen concentration and arterial oxygen saturation.

Ventilation

Most newly born infants who require positive-pressure ventilation can be adequately ventilated with a bag and mask. Indications for positive-pressure ventilation include apnea or gasping respirations, heart rate <100 bpm, and persistent central cyanosis despite 100% oxygen.

Although the pressure required for establishment of air breathing is variable and unpredictable, higher inflation pressures (30 to 40 cm H_2O or higher) and longer inflation times may be required for the first several breaths than for subsequent breaths.[18,19] Visible chest expansion is a more reliable sign of appropriate inflation pressures than any specific manometer reading. The assisted ventilation rate should be 40 to 60 breaths per minute (30 breaths per minute when chest compressions are also being delivered). Signs of adequate ventilation include bilateral expansion of the lungs, as assessed by chest wall movement and breath sounds, and improvement in heart rate and color. If ventilation is inadequate, check the seal between mask and face, clear any airway obstruction (adjust head position, clear secretions, open the infant's mouth), and finally increase inflation pressure. Prolonged bag-mask ventilation may produce gastric inflation; this should be relieved by insertion of an 8F orogastric tube that is aspirated with a syringe and left open to air. If such maneuvers do not result in adequate ventilation, endotracheal intubation should follow.

After 30 seconds of adequate ventilation with 100% oxygen, spontaneous breathing and heart rate should be checked. If spontaneous respirations are present and the heart rate is ≥100 bpm, positive-pressure ventilation may be gradually reduced and discontinued. Gentle tactile stimulation may help maintain and improve spontaneous respirations while free-flow oxygen is administered. If spontaneous respirations are inadequate or if heart rate remains below 100 bpm, assisted ventilation must continue with bag and mask or tracheal tube. If the heart rate is <60 bpm, continue assisted ventilation, begin chest compressions, and consider endotracheal intubation.

The key to successful neonatal resuscitation is establishment of adequate ventilation. Reversal of hypoxia, acidosis, and bradycardia depends on adequate inflation of fluid-filled lungs with air or oxygen.[44,45] Although 100% oxygen has been used traditionally for rapid reversal of hypoxia, there is biochemical evidence and preliminary clinical evidence to argue for resuscitation with lower oxygen concentrations.[46-48] Current clinical data, however, is insufficient to justify adopting this as routine practice. If assisted ventilation is required, deliver 100% oxygen by positive-pressure ventilation. If supplemental oxygen is unavailable, initiate resuscitation of the newly born infant with positive-pressure ventilation and room air (Class Indeterminate, LOE 2).

Ventilation Bags

Resuscitation bags used for neonates should be no larger than 750 mL; larger bag volumes make it difficult to judge delivery of the small tidal volumes (5 to 8 mL/kg) that newly born infants require. Bags for neonatal resuscitation can be either self-inflating or flow-inflating.

Self-Inflating Bags

The self-inflating bag refills independently of gas flow because of the recoil of the bag. To permit rapid reinflation, most bags of this type have an intake valve at one end that pulls in room air, diluting the oxygen flowing into the bag at a fixed rate. Delivery of high concentrations of oxygen (90% to 100%) with a self-inflating bag requires an attached oxygen reservoir.

To maintain inflation pressure for at least 1 second,

a minimum bag volume of 450 to 500 mL may be necessary. If the device contains a pressure-release valve, it should release at approximately 30 to 35 cm H_2O pressure and should have an override feature to permit delivery of higher pressures if necessary to achieve good chest expansion. Self-inflating bags that are not pressure-limited or that have a device to bypass the pressure-release valve should be equipped with an in-line manometer. Do not use self-inflating bags to deliver oxygen passively through the mask because the flow of oxygen is unreliable unless the bag is being squeezed.

Flow-Inflating Bags

The flow-inflating (anesthesia) bag inflates only when compressed gas is flowing into it and the patient outlet is at least partially occluded. Proper use requires adjustment of the flow of gas into the gas inlet, adjustment of the flow of gas out through the flow-control valve, and creation of a tight seal between the mask and face. Because a flow-inflating bag is capable of delivering very high pressures, a manometer should be connected to the bag to monitor peak and end-expiratory pressures. More training is required for proper use of the flow-inflating bag than the self-inflating bag,[49] but the flow-inflating bag can provide a greater range of peak inspiratory pressures and more reliable control of oxygen concentration. High concentrations of oxygen may be delivered passively through the mask of a flow-inflating bag.

Face Masks

Masks should be of appropriate size to seal around the mouth and nose but not cover the eyes or overlap the chin. A range of sizes should be available. A round mask can seal effectively on the face of a small infant; anatomically shaped masks better fit the contours of a large term infant's face. Masks should be designed to have low dead space (<5 mL). A mask with a cushioned rim is preferable to one without because the cushioned rim facilitates creation of a tight seal without exerting excessive pressure on the face.[50]

Laryngeal Mask Airway Ventilation

Masks that fit over the laryngeal inlet have been shown to be effective for ventilating newly born full-term infants.[51] There is limited data on the use of these devices in small preterm infants,[52] however, and their use in the setting of meconium-stained amniotic fluid has not been studied. The laryngeal mask airway, when used by appropriately trained providers, may be an effective alternative for establishing an airway in resuscitation of the newly born infant, especially in the case of ineffective bag-mask ventilation or failed endotracheal intubation (Class Indeterminate, LOE 5). However, we cannot recommend routine use of the laryngeal mask airway at this time, and the device cannot replace endotracheal intubation for meconium suctioning.

Endotracheal Intubation

Endotracheal intubation may be indicated at several points during neonatal resuscitation:

- When tracheal suctioning for meconium is required
- If bag-mask ventilation is ineffective or prolonged
- When chest compressions are performed
- When tracheal administration of medications is desired
- Special resuscitation circumstances, such as congenital diaphragmatic hernia or extremely low birth weight

The timing of endotracheal intubation may also depend on the skill and experience of the resuscitator.

Keep the supplies and equipment for endotracheal intubation together and readily available in each delivery room, nursery, and Emergency Department. Preferred tracheal tubes have a uniform diameter (without a shoulder) and have a natural curve, a radiopaque indicator line, and markings to indicate the appropriate depth of insertion. If a stylet is used, it must not protrude beyond the tip of the tube. Table 3 provides a guideline for selection of tracheal tube sizes and depths of insertion. Positioning the vocal cord guide (a line proximal to the tip of the tube) at the level of the vocal cords should position the tip of the tube above the carina. Proper depth of insertion can also be estimated by calculating the depth at the lips according to the following formula:

$$\text{weight in kilograms} + 6 \text{ cm}$$
$$= \text{insertion depth at lip in cm}$$

Perform endotracheal intubation orally, using a laryngoscope with a straight blade (size 0 for premature infants, size 1 for term infants). Insert the tip of the laryngoscope into the vallecula or onto the epiglottis and elevate gently to reveal the vocal cords. Cricoid pressure may be helpful. Insert the tube to an appropriate depth through the vocal cords as indicated by the vocal cord guide line and check its position by the centimeter marking at the upper lip. Record and maintain this depth of insertion. Variation in head position will alter the depth of insertion and may predispose to unintentional extubation or endobronchial intubation.[53,54]

After endotracheal intubation, confirm the position of the tube by the following:

- Observing symmetrical chest-wall motion
- Listening for equal breath sounds, especially in the axillae, and for absence of breath sounds over the stomach
- Confirming absence of gastric inflation
- Watching for a fog of moisture in the tube during exhalation
- Noting improvement in heart rate, color, and activity of the infant

An exhaled-CO_2 monitor may be used to verify tracheal tube placement.[55] These devices are associated with some false-negative but few false-positive results.[56] Monitoring of exhaled CO_2 can be useful in the secondary confirmation of tracheal intubation in the newly born, particularly when clinical assessment is equivocal (Class Indeterminate, LOE 5). Data about sensitivity and specificity of exhaled CO_2 detectors in reflecting tracheal tube position is limited in newly born infants. Extrapolation of data from other age groups is problematic because conditions common to the newborn period, including inadequate pulmonary expansion, decreased pulmonary blood flow, and small tidal volumes, may influence the interpretation of the exhaled CO_2 concentration.

Chest Compressions

Asphyxia causes peripheral vasoconstriction, tissue hypoxia, acidosis, poor myocardial contractility, bradycardia, and eventually cardiac arrest. Establishment of adequate ventilation and oxygenation will restore vital signs in the vast majority of newly born infants. In deciding when to initiate chest compressions, consider the heart rate, the change of heart rate, and the time elapsed after initiation of resuscitative measures. Because chest compressions may diminish the effectiveness of ventilation, do not initiate them until lung inflation and ventilation have been established.

The general indication for initiation of chest compressions is a heart rate <60 bpm despite adequate ventilation with 100% oxygen for 30 seconds. Although it has been common practice to give compressions if the heart rate is 60 to 80 bpm and the heart rate is not rising, ventilation should be the priority in resuscitation of the newly born. Provision of chest compressions is likely to compete with provision of effective ventilation. Because no scientific data suggests an evidence-based resolution, the ILCOR Working Group recommends that compressions be initiated for a heart rate of <60 bpm based on construct validity (ease of teaching and skill retention).

Compression Technique

Compressions should be delivered on the lower third of the sternum.[57,58] Acceptable techniques are (1) 2 thumbs on the sternum, superimposed or adjacent to each other according to the size of the infant, with fingers encircling the chest and supporting the back (the 2 thumb–encircling hands technique), and (2) 2 fingers placed on the sternum at right angles to the chest with the other hand supporting the back.[59-61] Data suggests that the 2 thumb–encircling hands technique may offer some advantages in generating peak systolic and coronary perfusion pressure and that providers prefer this technique to the 2-finger technique.[59-63] For this reason, we prefer the

TABLE 3. Suggested Tracheal Tube Size and Depth of Insertion According to Weight and Gestational Age

Weight, g	Gestational Age, wk	Tube Size, mm (ID)	Depth of Insertion From Upper Lip, cm
<1000	<28	2.5	6.5–7
1000–2000	28–34	3.0	7–8
2000–3000	34–38	3.5	8–9
>3000	>38	3.5–4.0	>9

ID indicates inner diameter.

2 thumb–encircling hands technique for healthcare providers performing chest compressions in newly born infants and older infants whose size permits its use (Class IIb, LOE 5).

Consensus of the ILCOR Working Group supports a relative rather than absolute depth of compression (ie, compress to approximately one third of the anterior-posterior diameter of the chest) to generate a palpable pulse. The pediatric basic life support guidelines recommend a relative compression depth of one third to one half of the anterior-posterior dimension of the chest. In the absence of specific data about ideal compression depth, these guidelines recommend compression to approximately one third the depth of the chest, but the compression depth must be adequate to produce a palpable pulse. Deliver compressions smoothly. A compression to relaxation ratio with a slightly shorter compression than relaxation phase offers theoretical advantages for blood flow in the very young infant.[64] Keep the thumbs or fingers on the sternum during the relaxation phase.

Coordinate compressions and ventilations to avoid simultaneous delivery.[65] There should be a 3:1 ratio of compressions to ventilations, with 90 compressions and 30 breaths to achieve approximately 120 events per minute. Thus, each event will be allotted approximately 1/2 second, with exhalation occurring during the first compression following each ventilation. Reassess the heart rate approximately every 30 seconds. Continue chest compressions until the spontaneous heart rate is ≥60 bpm.

MEDICATIONS

Drugs are rarely indicated in resuscitation of the newly born infant.[66] Bradycardia in the newly born infant is usually the result of inadequate lung inflation or profound hypoxia, and adequate ventilation is the most important step in correcting bradycardia. Administer medications if, despite adequate ventilation with 100% oxygen and chest compressions, the heart rate remains <60 bpm.

Medications and Volume Expansion

Epinephrine

Administration of epinephrine is indicated when the heart rate remains <60 bpm after a minimum of 30 seconds of adequate ventilation and chest compressions (Class I). Epinephrine is particularly indicated in the presence of asystole.

Epinephrine has both α- and β-adrenergic–stimulating properties; however, in cardiac arrest, α-adrenergic–mediated vasoconstriction may be the more important action.[67] Vasoconstriction elevates the perfusion pressure during chest compression, enhancing delivery of oxygen to the heart and brain.[68] Epinephrine also enhances the contractile state of the heart, stimulates spontaneous contractions, and increases heart rate.

The recommended intravenous or endotracheal dose is 0.1 to 0.3 mL/kg of a 1:10 000 solution (0.01 to 0.03 mg/kg), repeated every 3 to 5 minutes as indicated. The data regarding effects of high-dose epinephrine for resuscitation of newly born infants is inadequate to support routine use of higher doses of epinephrine (Class Indeterminate, LOE 4). Higher doses have been associated with exaggerated hypertension but lower cardiac output in animals.[69,70] The sequence of hypotension followed by hypertension likely increases the risk of intracranial hemorrhage, especially in preterm infants.[71]

Volume Expanders

Volume expanders may be necessary to resuscitate a newly born infant who is hypovolemic. Suspect hypovolemia in any infant who fails to respond to resuscitation. Consider volume expansion when there has been suspected blood loss or the infant appears to be in shock (pale, poor perfusion, weak pulse) and has not responded adequately to other resuscitative measures (Class I). The fluid of choice for volume expansion is an isotonic crystalloid solution such as normal saline or Ringer's lactate (Class IIb, LOE 7). Administration of O-negative red blood cells may be indicated for replacement of large-volume blood loss (Class IIb, LOE 7). Albumin-containing solutions are less frequently used for initial volume expansion because of limited availability, risk of infectious disease, and an observed association with increased mortality.[72]

The initial dose of volume expander is 10 mL/kg given by slow intravenous push over 5 to 10 minutes. The dose may be repeated after further clinical assessment and observation of response. Higher bolus volumes have been recommended for resuscitation of older infants. However, volume overload or complications such as intracranial hemorrhage may result from inappropriate intravascular volume expansion in asphyxiated newly born infants as well as in preterm infants.[73,74]

Bicarbonate

There is insufficient data to recommend routine use of bicarbonate in resuscitation of the newly born. In fact, the hyperosmolarity and CO_2-generating properties of sodium bicarbonate may be detrimental to myocardial or cerebral function.[75–77] Use of sodium bicarbonate is discouraged during brief CPR. If it is used during prolonged arrests unresponsive to other therapy, it should be given only after establishment of adequate ventilation and circulation.[78] Later use of bicarbonate for treatment of persistent metabolic acidosis or hyperkalemia should be directed by arterial blood gas levels or serum chemistries, among other evaluations. A dose of 1 to 2 mEq/kg of a 0.5 mEq/mL solution may be given by slow intravenous push (over at least 2 minutes) after adequate ventilation and perfusion have been established.

Naloxone

Naloxone hydrochloride is a narcotic antagonist without respiratory-depressant activity. It is specifically indicated for reversal of respiratory depression in a newly born infant whose mother received narcotics within 4 hours of delivery. Always establish and maintain adequate ventilation before administration of naloxone. Do not administer naloxone to newly born infants whose mothers are suspected of having recently abused narcotic drugs because it may precipitate abrupt withdrawal signs in such infants.

The recommended dose of naloxone is 0.1 mg/kg of a 0.4 mg/mL or 1.0 mg/mL solution given intravenously, endotracheally, or—if perfusion is adequate—intramuscularly or subcutaneously. Because the duration of action of narcotics may exceed that of naloxone, continued monitoring of respiratory function is essential, and repeated naloxone doses may be necessary to prevent recurrent apnea.

Routes of Medication Administration

The tracheal route is generally the most rapidly accessible route for drug administration during resuscitation. It may be used for administration of epinephrine and naloxone, but it should not be used during resuscitation for administration of caustic agents such as sodium bicarbonate. The tracheal route of administration may result in a more variable response to epinephrine than the intravenous route[79-81]; however, neonatal data is insufficient to recommend a higher dose of epinephrine for tracheal administration.

Attempt to establish intravenous access in neonates who fail to respond to tracheally administered epinephrine. The umbilical vein is the most rapidly accessible venous route; it may be used for epinephrine or naloxone administration as well as for administration of volume expanders and bicarbonate. Insert a 3.5F or 5F radiopaque catheter so that the tip is just below skin level and a free flow of blood returns on aspiration. Deep insertion poses the risk of infusion of hypertonic and vasoactive medications into the liver. Take care to avoid introduction of air emboli into the umbilical vein.

Peripheral sites for venous access (scalp or peripheral vein) may be adequate but are usually more difficult to cannulate. Naloxone may be given intramuscularly or subcutaneously but only after effective assisted ventilation has been established and only if the infant's peripheral circulation is adequate. We do not recommend administration of resuscitation drugs through the umbilical artery because the artery is often not rapidly accessible and complications may result if vasoactive or hypertonic drugs (eg, epinephrine or bicarbonate) are given by this route.

Intraosseous lines are not commonly used in newly born infants because the umbilical vein is more accessible, the small bones are fragile, and the intraosseous space is small in a premature infant. Intraosseous access has been shown to be useful in the neonate and older infant when vascular access is difficult to achieve.[82] Intraosseous access can be used as an alternative route for medication/volume expansion if umbilical or other direct venous access is not readily attainable (Class IIb, LOE 5).

SPECIAL RESUSCITATION CIRCUMSTANCES

Several circumstances have unique implications for resuscitation of the newly born infant. Prenatal diagnosis and certain features of the perinatal history and clinical course may alert the resuscitation team to these special circumstances. Meconium aspiration (see above), multiple birth, and prematurity are common conditions with immediate implications for the resuscitation team at delivery. Other circumstances that may affect opening of the airway, timing of endotracheal intubation, and selection and administration of volume expanders are presented in Table 4.

Prematurity

The incidence of perinatal depression is markedly increased among preterm neonates because of the complications associated with preterm labor and the physiological immaturity and lability of the preterm infant.[83] Diminished lung compliance, respiratory musculature, and respiratory drive may contribute to the need for assisted ventilation.

Some experts recommend early elective intubation of extremely preterm infants (eg, <28 weeks of ges-

TABLE 4.   Special Circumstances in Resuscitation of the Newly Born Infant

Condition	History/Clinical Signs	Actions
Mechanical blockage of the airway		
Meconium or mucus blockage	Meconium-stained amniotic fluid Poor chest wall movement	Intubation for suctioning/ventilation
Choanal atresia	Pink when crying, cyanotic when quiet	Oral airway Endotracheal intubation
Pharyngeal airway malformation	Persistent retractions, poor air entry	Prone positioning, posterior nasopharyngeal tube
Impaired lung function		
Pneumothorax	Asymmetrical breath sounds Persistent cyanosis/bradycardia	Needle thoracentesis
Pleural effusions/ascites	Diminished air movement Persistent cyanosis/bradycardia	Immediate intubation Needle thoracentesis, paracentesis Possible volume expansion
Congenital diaphragmatic hernia	Asymmetrical breath sounds Persistent cyanosis/bradycardia Scaphoid abdomen	Endotracheal intubation Placement of orogastric catheter
Pneumonia/sepsis	Diminished air movement Persistent cyanosis/bradycardia	Endotracheal intubation Possible volume expansion
Impaired cardiac function		
Congenital heart disease	Persistent cyanosis/bradycardia	Diagnostic evaluation
Fetal/maternal hemorrhage	Pallor; poor response to resuscitation	Volume expansion, possibly including red blood cells

tation) to help establish an air-fluid interface,[84] while others recommend that this be accomplished with oxygen administration via mask or nasal prongs.[85] Many infants younger than 30 to 31 weeks will undergo intubation for surfactant administration after the initial stages of resuscitation have been successful.[86]

A number of factors can complicate resuscitation of the premature infant. Because premature infants have low body fat and a high ratio of surface area to body mass, they are also more difficult to keep warm. Their immature brains and the presence of a fragile germinal matrix predispose them to development of intracranial hemorrhage after episodes of hypoxia or rapid changes in vascular pressure and osmolarity.[77,87,88] For this reason, avoid rapid boluses of volume expanders or hyperosmolar solutions.

Multiple Births

Multiple births are more frequently associated with a need for resuscitation because of abnormalities of placentation, compromise of cord blood flow, or mechanical complications during delivery. Monozygotic multiple fetuses may also have abnormalities of blood volume resulting from interfetal vascular anastomoses.

POSTRESUSCITATION ISSUES

Continuing Care of the Newly Born Infant
After Resuscitation

Supportive or ongoing care, monitoring, and appropriate diagnostic evaluation are required after resuscitation. Once adequate ventilation and circulation have been established, the infant is still at risk and should be maintained in or transferred to an environment in which close monitoring and anticipatory care can be provided. Postresuscitation monitoring should include monitoring of heart rate, respiratory rate, administered oxygen concentration, and arterial oxygen saturation, with blood gas analysis as indicated. Document blood pressure and check the blood glucose level during stabilization after resuscitation. Consider ongoing blood glucose screening and documentation of calcium. A chest radiograph may help elucidate underlying causes of the arrest or detect complications, such as pneumothorax. Additional postresuscitation care may include treatment of hypotension with volume expanders or pressors, treatment of possible infection or seizures, initiation of appropriate fluid therapy, and documentation of observations and actions.

Documentation of Resuscitation

Thorough documentation of assessments and resuscitative actions is essential for good clinical care, for communication, and for medicolegal concerns. The Apgar scores quantify and summarize the response of the newly born infant to the extrauterine environment and to resuscitation (Table 5).[89,90] Assign Apgar scores at 1 and 5 minutes after birth and then sequentially every 5 minutes until vital signs have stabilized. The Apgar scores should not dictate appropriate resuscitative actions, nor should interventions for depressed infants be delayed until the 1-minute assessment. Complete documentation must also include a narrative description of interventions performed and their timing.

Continuing Care of the Family

When time permits, the team responsible for care of the newly born should introduce themselves to the mother and family before delivery. They should outline the proposed plan of care and solicit the family's questions. Especially in cases of potentially lethal fetal malformations or extreme prematurity, the family should be asked to articulate their beliefs and desires about the extent of resuscitation, and the team should outline its planned approach (see below).

After delivery the mother continues to be a patient herself, with physical and emotional needs. The team caring for the newly born infant should inform the parents of the infant's condition at the earliest opportunity. If resuscitation is necessary, inform the parents of the procedures undertaken and their indications. Encourage the parents to ask questions, and answer their questions as frankly and honestly as possible. Make every effort to enable the parents to have contact with the newly born infant.

ETHICS

There are circumstances in which noninitiation or discontinuation of resuscitation in the delivery room may be appropriate. However, national and local protocols should dictate the procedures to be followed. Changes in resuscitation and intensive care practices and neonatal outcome make it imperative that all such protocols be reviewed regularly and modified as necessary.

Noninitiation of Resuscitation

The delivery of extremely immature infants and infants with severe congenital anomalies raises questions about initiation of resuscitation.[91-93] Noninitia-

TABLE 5.   Apgar Scoring

Sign	Score		
	0	1	2
Heart rate	Absent	Slow (<100 bpm)	≥100 bpm
Respirations	Absent	Slow, irregular	Good, crying
Muscle tone	Limp	Some flexion	Active motion
Reflex irritability (catheter in nares, tactile stimulation)	No response	Grimace	Cough, sneeze, cry
Color	Blue or pale	Pink body, blue extremities	Completely pink

bpm indicates beats per minute.

tion of resuscitation in the delivery room is appropriate for infants with confirmed gestation <23 weeks or birth weight <400 g, anencephaly, or confirmed trisomy 13 or 18. Current data suggests that resuscitation of these newly born infants is very unlikely to result in survival or survival without severe disability (Class IIb, LOE 5).[94,95] However, antenatal information may be incomplete or unreliable. In cases of uncertain prognosis, including uncertain gestational age, resuscitation options include a trial of therapy and noninitiation or discontinuation of resuscitation after assessment of the infant. In such cases, initiation of resuscitation at delivery does not mandate continued support.

Noninitiation of support and later withdrawal of support are generally considered to be ethically equivalent; however, the latter approach allows time to gather more complete clinical information and to provide counseling to the family. Ongoing evaluation and discussion with the parents and the healthcare team should guide continuation versus withdrawal of support. In general, there is no advantage to delayed, graded, or partial support; if the infant survives, outcome may be worsened as a result of this approach.

Discontinuation of Resuscitation

Discontinuation of resuscitative efforts may be appropriate if resuscitation of an infant with cardiorespiratory arrest does not result in spontaneous circulation in 15 minutes. Resuscitation of newly born infants after 10 minutes of asystole is very unlikely to result in survival or survival without severe disability (Class IIb, LOE 5).[96–99] We recommend local discussions to formulate guidelines consistent with local resources and outcome data.

CONTRIBUTORS AND REVIEWERS FOR THE NEONATAL RESUSCITATION GUIDELINES
Susan Niermeyer, MD, Editor
John Kattwinkel, MD
Patrick Van Reempts, MD
Vinay Nadkarni, MD
Barbara Phillips, MD
David Zideman, MD

Denis Azzopardi, MD
Robert Berg, MD
David Boyle, MD
Robert Boyle, MD
David Burchfield, MD
Waldemar Carlo, MD
Leon Chameides, MD
Susan Denson, MD
Mary Fallat, MD
Michael Gerardi, MD
Alistair Gunn, MD
Mary Fran Hazinski, MSN, RN
William Keenan, MD
Stefanie Knaebel, MD
Anthony Milner, MD
Jeffrey Perlman, MD
Ola Didrick Saugstad, MD
Charles Schleien, MD
Alfonso Solimano, MD
Michael Speer, MD

Suzanne Toce, MD
Thomas Wiswell, MD
Arno Zaritsky, MD

Reviewers:
1998–2000 members of the Neonatal Resuscitation Steering Committee of the American Academy of Pediatrics, the Pediatric Working Group of the International Liaison Committee on Resuscitation, and the Pediatric Resuscitation Subcommittee and Emergency Cardiovascular Care Committee of the American Heart Association.

REFERENCES

1. Saugstad OD. Practical aspects of resuscitating asphyxiated newborn infants. *Eur J Pediatr*. 1998;157(suppl 1):S11–S15.
2. Palme-Kilander C. Methods of resuscitation in low-Apgar-score newborn infants: a national survey. *Acta Paediatr*. 1992;81:739–744.
3. *World Health Report*. Geneva, Switzerland: World Health Organization; 1995.
4. Perlman JM, Risser R. Cardiopulmonary resuscitation in the delivery room: associated clinical events. *Arch Pediatr Adolesc Med*. 1995;149:20–25.
5. Cummins RO, Chamberlain DA, Abramson NS, et al. Recommended guidelines for uniform reporting of data from out-of-hospital cardiac arrest: the Utstein style. *Circulation*. 1991;84:960–975.
6. Cummins RO, Chamberlain DA, Hazinski MF, et al. Recommended guidelines for reviewing, reporting, and conducting research on in-hospital resuscitation: the in-hospital "Utstein style." *Circulation*. 1997; 95:2213–2239.
7. Zaritsky A, Nadkarni V, Hazinski MF, Foltin G, Quan L, Wright J, Fiser D, Zideman D, O'Malley P, Chameides L, Writing Group. Recommended guidelines for uniform reporting of pediatric advanced life support: the pediatric Utstein style: a statement for healthcare professionals from a task force of the American Academy of Pediatrics, the American Heart Association, and the European Resuscitation Council. *Circulation*. 1995;92:2006–2020.
8. Idris AH, Becker LB, Ornato JP, Hedges JR, Bircher NG, Chandra NC, Cummins RO, Dick W, Ebmeyer U, Halperin HR, Hazinski MF, Kerber RE, Kern KB, Safar P, Steen PA, Swindle MM, Tsitlik JE, von Planta I, von Planta M, Wears RL, Weil MH, Writing Group. Utstein-style guidelines for uniform reporting of laboratory CPR research: a statement for healthcare professionals from a task force of the American Heart Association, the American College of Emergency Physicians, the American College of Cardiology, the European Resuscitation Council, the Heart and Stroke Foundation of Canada, the Institute of Critical Care Medicine, the Safar Center for Resuscitation Research, and the Society for Academic Emergency Medicine. *Circulation*. 1996;94:2324–2336.
9. Nadkarni V, Hazinski MF, Zideman D, Kattwinkel J, Quan L, Bingham R, Zaritsky A, Bland J, Kramer E, Tiballs J. Paediatric life support: an advisory statement by the Paediatric Life Support Working Group of the International Liaison Committee on Resuscitation. *Resuscitation*. 1997;34:115–127.
10. Kattwinkel J, Niermeyer S, Nadkarni V, Tibballs J, Phillips B, Zideman D, Van Reempts P, Osmond M. ILCOR advisory statement: resuscitation of the newly born infant: an advisory statement from the pediatric working group of the International Liaison Committee on Resuscitation. *Circulation*. 1999;99:1927–1938.
11. Guidelines for cardiopulmonary resuscitation and emergency cardiac care: Emergency Cardiac Care Committee and Subcommittees, American Heart Association, part V: pediatric basic life support [see comments]. *JAMA*. 1992;268:2251–2261.
12. Bloom RS, Cropley C, AHA/AAP Neonatal Resuscitation Program Steering Committee, American Heart Association. American Academy of Pediatrics. Textbook of Neonatal Resuscitation/Ronald S. Bloom, Catherine Cropley, and the AHA/AAP Neonatal Resuscitation Program Steering Committee [Rev. ed.];1 v. (various pagings): ill.; 28 cm. Elk Grove Village, IL: American Academy of Pediatrics: American Heart Association; 1994.
13. Kloeck WGJ, Kramer E. Resuscitation Council of Southern Africa: new recommendations for BLS in adults, children and infants. *Trauma Emerg Med*. 1997;14:13–31, 40–67.
14. Advanced Life Support Committee of the Australian Resuscitation Council. Paediatric advanced life support: Australian Resuscitation

Council guidelines: Advanced Life Support Committee of the Australian Resuscitation Council. *Med J Aust.* 1996;165:199–201, 204–206.

15. European Resuscitation Council. Pediatric basic life support: to be read in conjunction with the International Liaison Committee on Resuscitation Pediatric Working Group Advisory Statement (April 1997). *Resuscitation.* 1998;37:97–100.

16. European Resuscitation Council. Pediatric advanced life support: to be read in conjunction with the International Liaison Committee on Resuscitation Pediatric Working Group Advisory Statement (April 1997). *Resuscitation.* 1998;37:101–102.

17. European Resuscitation Council. Recommendations on resuscitation of babies at birth: to be read in conjunction with the International Liaison Committee on Resuscitation Pediatric Working Group Advisory Statement (April 1997). *Resuscitation.* 1998;37:103–110.

18. Vyas H, Milner AD, Hopkin IE, Boon AW. Physiologic responses to prolonged slow-rise inflation in the resuscitation of the asphyxiated newborn infant. *J Pediatr.* 1981;99:635–639.

19. Vyas H, Field D, Milner AD, Hopkin IE. Determinants of the first inspiratory volume and functional residual capacity at birth. *Pediatr Pulmonol.* 1986;2:189–193.

20. Jobe A. The respiratory system. In: Fanaroff AA, Martin RJ, et al, eds. *Neonatal Perinatal Medicine.* St Louis, Mo: CV Mosby; 1997:991–1018.

21. Gregory GA, Gooding CA, Phibbs RH, Tooley WH. Meconium aspiration in infants: a prospective study. *J Pediatr.* 1974;85:848–852.

22. Peliowski A, Finer NN. Birth asphyxia in the term infant. In: Sinclair JC, Bracken MB, et al, eds. *Effective Care of the Newborn Infant.* Oxford, UK: Oxford University Press; 1992:249–273.

23. Dawes GF. *Fetal and Neonatal Physiology: A Comparative Study of the Changes at Birth.* Chicago, Ill: Year Book Medical Publishers; 1968: 149–151.

24. Whitelaw CC, Goldsmith LJ. Comparison of two techniques for determining the presence of a pulse in an infant [letter]. *Acad Emerg Med.* 1997;4:153–154.

25. Theophilopoulos DT, Burchfield DJ. Accuracy of different methods for heart rate determination during simulated neonatal resuscitations. *J Perinatol.* 1998;18:65–67.

26. Gandy GM, Adamson SK Jr, Cunningham N, Silverman WA, James LS. Thermal environment and acid-base homeostasis in human infants during the first few hours of life. *J Clin Invest.* 1964;43:751–758.

27. Dahm LS, James LS. Newborn temperature and calculated heat loss in the delivery room. *Pediatrics.* 1972;49:504–513.

28. Perlman JM. Maternal fever and neonatal depression: preliminary observations. *Clin Pediatr.* 1999;38:287–291.

29. Lieberman E, Lang J, Richardson DK, Frigoletto FD, Heffner LJ, Cohen A. Intrapartum maternal fever and neonatal outcome. *Pediatrics.* 2000; 105:8–13.

30. Vannucci RC, Perlman JM. Interventions for perinatal hypoxic-ischemic encephalopathy [see comments]. *Pediatrics.* 1997;100:1004–1014.

31. Edwards AD, Wyatt JS, Thoreson M. Treatment of hypoxic-ischemic brain damage by moderate hypothermia. *Arch Dis Child Fetal Neonatal Ed.* 1998;78:F85–F88.

32. Gunn AJ, Gluckman PD, Gunn TR. Selective head cooling in newborn infants after perinatal asphyxia: a safety study [see comments]. *Pediatrics.* 1998;102:885–892.

33. Estol PC, Piriz H, Basalo S, Simini F, Grela C. Oro-naso-pharyngeal suction at birth: effects on respiratory adaptation of normal term vaginally born infants. *J Perinatal Med.* 1992;20:297–305.

34. Cordero L Jr, Hon EH. Neonatal bradycardia following nasopharyngeal stimulation. *J Pediatr.* 1971;78:441–447.

35. Wiswell TE, Tuggle JM, Turner BS. Meconium aspiration syndrome: have we made a difference? [see comments]. *Pediatrics.* 1990;85:715–721.

36. Carson BS, Losey RW, Bowes WA Jr, Simmons MA. Combined obstetric and pediatric approach to prevent meconium aspiration syndrome. *Am J Obstet Gynecol.* 1976;126:712–715.

37. Locus P, Yeomans E, Crosby U. Efficacy of bulb versus DeLee suction at deliveries complicated by meconium stained amniotic fluid [see comments]. *Am J Perinatol.* 1990;7:87–91.

38. Rossi EM, Philipson EH, Williams TG, Kalhan SC. Meconium aspiration syndrome: intrapartum and neonatal attributes [see comments]. *Am J Obstet Gynecol.* 1989;161:1106–1110.

39. Falciglia HS. Failure to prevent meconium aspiration syndrome. *Obstet Gynecol.* 1988;71:349–353.

40. Greenough A. Meconium aspiration syndrome: prevention and treatment. *Early Hum Dev.* 1995;41:183–192.

41. Wiswell TE, Bent RC. Meconium staining and the meconium aspiration syndrome: unresolved issues. *Pediatr Clin North Am.* 1993;40:955–981.

42. Wiswell TE. Meconium in the Delivery Room Trial Group: delivery room management of the apparently vigorous meconium-stained

43. Linder N, Aranda JV, Tsur M, et al. Need for endotracheal intubation and suction in meconium-stained neonates. *J Pediatr.* 1988;112:613–615.

44. de Burgh Daly M, Angell-James JE, Elsner R. Role of carotid-body chemoreceptors and their reflex interactions in bradycardia and cardiac arrest. *Lancet.* 1979;1:764–767.

45. de Burgh Daly M. Interactions between respiration and circulation. In: Cherniack NS, Widdicombe JG, eds. *Handbook of Physiology, Section 3, The Respiratory System.* Bethesda, Md: American Physiological Society; 1986:529–595.

46. Rootwelt T, Odden J, Hall C, Ganes T, Saugstad OD. Cerebral blood flow and evoked potentials during reoxygenation with 21 or 100% O_2 in newborn pigs. *J Appl Physiol.* 1993;75:2054–2060.

47. Ramji S, Ahuja S, Thirupuram S, Rootwelt T, Rooth G, Saugstad OD. Resuscitation of asphyxic newborn infants with room air or 100% oxygen. *Pediatr Res.* 1993;34:809–812.

48. Saugstad OD, Rootwelt T, Aalen O. Resuscitation of asphyxiated newborn infants with room air or oxygen: an international controlled trial: the Resair 2 Study. *Pediatrics.* 1998;102:e1.

49. Kanter RK. Evaluation of mask-bag ventilation in resuscitation of infants. *Am J Dis Child.* 1987;141:761–763.

50. Palme C, Nystrom B, Tunell R. An evaluation of the efficiency of face masks in the resuscitation of newborn infants. *Lancet.* 1985;1:207–210.

51. Paterson SJ, Byrne PJ, Molesky MG, Seal RF, Finucane BT. Neonatal resuscitation using the laryngeal mask airway [see comments]. *Anesthesiology.* 1994;80:1248–1253, discussion 27A.

52. Gandini D, Brimacombe JR. Neonatal resuscitation with the laryngeal mask airway in normal and low birth weight infants. *Anesth Analg.* 1999;89:642–643.

53. Todres ID, deBros F, Kramer SS, Moylan FM, Shannon DC. Endotracheal tube displacement in the newborn infant. *J Pediatr.* 1976;89: 126–127.

54. Rotschild A, Chitayat D, Puterman ML, Phang MS, Ling E, Baldwin V. Optimal positioning of endotracheal tubes for ventilation of preterm infants. *Am J Dis Child.* 1991;145:1007–1012.

55. Aziz HF, Martin JB, Moore JJ. The pediatric end-tidal carbon dioxide detector role in endotracheal intubation in newborns. *J Perinatol.* 1999; 19:110–113.

56. Bhende MS, Thompson AE, Orr RA. Utility of an end-tidal carbon dioxide detector during stabilization and transport of critically ill children. *Pediatrics.* 1992;89:1042–1044.

57. Orlowski JP. Optimum position for external cardiac compression in infants and young children. *Ann Emerg Med.* 1986;15:667–673.

58. Phillips GW, Zideman DA. Relation of infant heart to sternum: its significance in cardiopulmonary resuscitation. *Lancet.* 1986;1:1024–1025.

59. Thaler MM, Stobie GHC. An improved technic of external cardiac compression in infants and young children. *N Engl J Med.* 1963;269: 606–610.

60. David R. Closed chest cardiac massage in the newborn infant. *Pediatrics.* 1988;81:552–554.

61. Todres ID, Rogers MC. Methods of external cardiac massage in the newborn infant. *J Pediatr.* 1975;86:781–782.

62. Menegazzi JJ, Auble TE, Nicklas KA, Hosack GM, Rack L, Goode JS. Two-thumb versus two-finger chest compression during CPR in a swine infant model of cardiac arrest [see comments]. *Ann Emerg Med.* 1993;22: 240–243.

63. Houri PK, Frank LR, Menegazzi JJ, Taylor R. A randomized, controlled trial of two-thumb vs two-finger chest compression in a swine infant model of cardiac arrest [see comment]. *Prehosp Emerg Care.* 1997;1: 65–67.

64. Dean JM, Koehler RC, Schleien CL, Berkowitz I, Michael JR, Atchison D, Rogers MC, Traystman RJ. Age-related effects of compression rate and duration in cardiopulmonary resuscitation. *J Appl Physiol.* 1990;68: 554–560.

65. Berkowitz ID, Chantarojanasiri T, Koehler RC, Schleien CL, Dean JM, Michael JR, Rogers MC, Traystman RJ. Blood flow during cardiopulmonary resuscitation with simultaneous compression and ventilation in infant pigs. *Pediatr Res.* 1989;26:558–564.

66. Burchfield DJ. Medication use in neonatal resuscitation. *Clin Perinatol.* 1999;26:683–691.

67. Zaritsky A, Chernow B. Use of catecholamines in pediatrics. *J Pediatr.* 1984;105:341–350.

68. Berkowitz ID, Gervais H, Schleien CL, Koehler RC, Dean JM, Traystman RJ. Epinephrine dosage effects on cerebral and myocardial blood flow in an infant swine model of cardiopulmonary resuscitation. *Anesthesiology.* 1991;75:1041–1050.

69. Berg RA, Otto CW, Kern KB, Hilwig RW, Sanders AB, Henry CP, Ewy

GA. A randomized, blinded trial of high-dose epinephrine versus standard-dose epinephrine in a swine model of pediatric asphyxial cardiac arrest. *Crit Care Med.* 1996;24:1695–1700.

70. Burchfield DJ, Preziosi MP, Lucas VW, Fan J. Effect of graded doses of epinephrine during asphyxia-induced bradycardia in newborn lambs. *Resuscitation.* 1993;25:235–244.

71. Pasternak JF, Groothuis DR, Fischer JM, Fischer DP. Regional cerebral blood flow in the beagle puppy model of neonatal intraventricular hemorrhage: studies during systemic hypertension. *Neurology.* 1983;33:559–566.

72. Cochrane Injuries Group Albumin Reviewers. Human albumin administration in critically ill patients: systematic review of randomised controlled trials. *BMJ.* 1998;317:235–240.

73. Usher R, Lind J. Blood volume of the newborn premature infant. *Acta Paediatr Scand.* 1965;54:419–431.

74. Funato M, Tamai H, Noma K, et al. Clinical events in association with timing of intraventricular hemorrhage in preterm infants. *J Pediatr.* 1992;121:614–619.

75. Kette F, Weil MH, von Planta M, Gazmuri RJ, Rackow EC. Buffer agents do not reverse intramyocardial acidosis during cardiac resuscitation. *Circulation.* 1990;81:1660–1666.

76. Kette F, Weil MH, Gazmuri RJ. Buffer solutions may compromise cardiac resuscitation by reducing coronary perfusion pressure [published correction appears in *JAMA.* 1991;266:3286] [See comments]. *JAMA.* 1991;266:2121–2126.

77. Papile LA, Burstein J, Burstein R, Koffler H, Koops B. Relationship of intravenous sodium bicarbonate infusions and cerebral intraventricular hemorrhage. *J Pediatr.* 1978;93:834–836.

78. Hein HA. The use of sodium bicarbonate in neonatal resuscitation: help or harm? *Pediatrics.* 1993;91:496–497.

79. Lindemann R. Resuscitation of the newborn: endotracheal administration of epinephrine. *Acta Paediatr Scand.* 1984;73:210–212.

80. Lucas VW, Preziosi MP, Burchfield DJ. Epinephrine absorption following endotracheal administration: effects of hypoxia-induced low pulmonary blood flow. *Resuscitation.* 1994;27:31–34.

81. Mullett CJ, Kong JQ, Romano JT, Polak MJ. Age-related changes in pulmonary venous epinephrine concentration and pulmonary vascular response after intratracheal epinephrine. *Pediatr Res.* 1992;31:458–461.

82. Ellemunter H, Simma B, Trawoger R, Maurer H. Intraosseous lines in preterm and full term neonates. *Arch Dis Child Fetal Neonatal Ed.* 1999;80:F74–F75.

83. MacDonald HM, Mulligan JC, Allen AC, Taylor PM. Neonatal asphyxia, I: relationship of obstetric and neonatal complications to neonatal mortality in 38,405 consecutive deliveries. *J Pediatr.* 1980;96:898–902.

84. Poets CF, Sens B. Changes in intubation rates and outcome of very low birth weight infants: a population study. *Pediatrics.* 1996;98:24–27.

85. Avery ME, Tooley WH, Keller JB, et al. Is chronic lung disease in low birth weight infants preventable? a survey of eight centers. *Pediatrics.* 1987;79:26–30.

86. Kattwinkel J. Surfactant: evolving issues. *Clin Perinatol.* 1998;25:17–32.

87. Simmons MA, Adcock EW III, Bard H, Battaglia FC. Hypernatremia and intracranial hemorrhage in neonates. *N Engl J Med.* 1974;291:6–10.

88. Hambleton G, Wigglesworth JS. Origin of intraventricular haemorrhage in the preterm infant. *Arch Dis Child.* 1976;51:651–659.

89. Apgar V, James LS. Further observations of the newborn scoring system. *Am J Dis Child.* 1962;104:419–428.

90. Chamberlain G, Banks J. Assessment of the Apgar score. *Lancet.* 1974;2:1225–1228.

91. Byrne PJ, Tyebkhan JM, Laing LM. Ethical decision-making and neonatal resuscitation. *Semin Perinatol.* 1994;18:36–41.

92. Davies JM, Reynolds BM. The ethics of cardiopulmonary resuscitation, I: background to decision making. *Arch Dis Child.* 1992;67:1498–1501.

93. Landwirth J. Ethical issues in pediatric and neonatal resuscitation. *Ann Emerg Med.* 1993;22:502–507.

94. Tyson JE, Younes N, Verter J, Wright LL. Viability, morbidity, and resource use among newborns of 501- to 800-g birth weight: National Institute of Child Health and Human Development Neonatal Research Network. *JAMA.* 1996;276:1645–1651.

95. Finer NN, Horbar JD, Carpenter JH. Cardiopulmonary resuscitation in the very low birth weight infant: the Vermont Oxford Network experience. *Pediatrics.* 1999;104:428–434.

96. Davis DJ. How aggressive should delivery room cardiopulmonary resuscitation be for extremely low birth weight neonates? [See comments]. *Pediatrics.* 1993;92:447–450.

97. Jain L, Ferre C, Vidyasagar D, Nath S, Sheftel D. Cardiopulmonary resuscitation of apparently stillborn infants: survival and long-term outcome [see comments]. *J Pediatr.* 1991;118:778–782.

98. Yeo CL, Tudehope DI. Outcome of resuscitated apparently stillborn infants: a ten year review. *J Paediatr Child Health.* 1994;30:129–133.

99. Casalaz DM, Marlow N, Speidel BD. Outcome of resuscitation following unexpected apparent stillbirth. *Arch Dis Child Fetal Neonatal Ed.* 1998;78:F112–F115.

Index

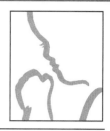

Index

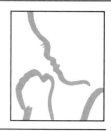

procedures to check before assisting ventilation with, 3-22

safety features of, 3-16

strength in squeezing the bag, 3-24–3-25

type available at hospital, 3-9

types available, 3-4–3-5

Resuscitation flow diagram, 1-8–1-11

Robin syndrome, 7-6

Routine care after resuscitation, 1-15

S

Seal, inadequacy of, as problem in bag-and-mask resuscitation, 3-26

Secondary apnea, 1-7

Seizures, 7-14

post-resuscitation care and, 7-16

Self-inflating resuscitation bags, 3-4, 3-5, 3-16, App. 9

advantages and disadvantages of, 3-6

controlling oxygen and pressure in, 3-14–3-15

general characteristics of, 3-7

parts of, 3-13

testing, 3-20

Shock, newborns in, 6-10

Shoulder roll in positioning of newborn, 2-7

Sodium bicarbonate, App. 11

administration of, through endotracheal tube, 6-5

metabolic acidosis and, 6-3, 6-12

Spontaneous respirations, failure of newborn to respond to, 7-3

Stylet, placement of, through endotracheal tube, 5-6

Suction equipment, need for, in neonatal resuscitation, 1-18

Suctioning, App. 8

Supportive care after resuscitation, 1-15

Surfactant administration as indication for endotracheal intubation, 5-2

Surfactant deficiency, post-resuscitation care and, 7-16

Suspected diaphragmatic hernia as indication for endotracheal intubation, 5-2

Syndrome of inappropriate antidiuretic hormone secretion (SIADH), 7-14

Systemic hypotension, 1-6

T

Tactile stimulation

and delay in resuscitation, 2-18

forms of

in assisting breathing in baby, 2-12

as hazardous, 2-13

of newborn, 2-12, App. 8

Temperature management, 7-15

neonatal resuscitation and, App. 2–3

and resuscitation for babies born out of hospital, 7-23

Thermoregulation after resuscitation, 1-15

Thrombocytopenia, post-resuscitation care and, 7-16

Thumb technique, position of hands using chest compressions, 4-6–4-7

Tongue, contusion or laceration of, as complication in endotracheal intubation, 5-24

Trachea, 5-8

length of, in premature newborn, 5-4

perforation of, as complication in endotracheal intubation, 5-24

suspicion that endotracheal intubation not in, 5-18

tip of endotracheal intubation located within, 5-19–5-20

Tracheal intubation, App. 3–4

Tracheal tube placement, confirmation of, App. 10

Transient tachypnea, post-resuscitation care and, 7-16

Transillumination of chest, 7-7

Transition

problems in, 1-6

response of baby to interruption in, 1-6–1-7

Two-finger technique, positioning of hands using, during chest compressions, 4-7

U

Umbilical vein, giving epinephrine through, 6-4, 6-6

Uncomplicated delivery, 2-2

V

Vallecula, 5-8

Valve assembly, 3-13

Vascular access

alternative route for, App. 3

and resuscitation for babies born out of hospital, 7-23

Ventilation, App. 2, App. 9. See also Bag-and-mask ventilation

bradycardic baby despite good, 7-10

coordination with, in chest compressions, 4-10

practice in, 4-11

cyanotic baby despite good, 7-10

and resuscitation for babies born out of hospital, 7-23

Ventilation bags. See Flow-inflating resuscitation bags; Self-inflating resuscitation bags

Vital signs, abnormal, 2-18

Vocal cord guide, 5-4

Vocal cords, 5-8

Volume expansion, 6-3, 6-11, App. 3, App. 11

choice for fluid for acute, App. 3